TABLE OF CONTENTS

INTRODUCTION

Did your New Year's resolution included something about losing weight or gaining more muscle? 2020 might be the year you hold on to those New Year's commitments, right? You will only have one glass of red wine right after this. That is a start. Right?

Do not panic. I have news for you before that guilt rolls in. What if I told you that there was a way to maintain your wine nights while moving on the path towards a healthy lifestyle? I promise, this is no joke.

Trendy new diets tend to crop up frequently, and one of the newest is the Sirtfood Diet. It has become a favorite for Europe's celebrities and is renowned for allowing red wine and chocolate to remain in one's diet. That is right. You can eat chocolate and drink your wine. Most notably, there is a theory that the Sirtfood Diet is the eating program behind Adele's weight loss transformation. Countries where people are now consuming a substantial amount of Sirtfoods as part of their conventional diet, like Japan and Italy, are ranked among the world's healthiest.

The Sirtfood diet first launched in 2016 and remains a hot topic in the dieting world. Founded by U.K. Health Specialists Aidan Goggins and Glen Matten, the Sirtfood Diet aims to activate the "skinny gene", or proteins belonging to the SIRT1 gene, to combat the symptoms of obesity, weight gain and aging. This protein is specifically known as sirtuin. Sirtuin proteins work to protect the cells within the body from detrimental stress while controlling inflammation, metabolism, and aging. These proteins are believed to affect the body 's capacity to lose fat and improve metabolism. However, some experts believe this is unlikely to be merely a fat loss but rather changes in skeletal muscle and liver glycogen stores.

Did you notice that the word food is in the diet name? Instead of promoting dwindling appetites and watching calorie consumption, the Sirtfood Diet is all about using 'wonder foods' to turbocharge your body. This not only maximizes weight reduction but can boost your general wellbeing in the long term. *How*? You may have heard of the word superfoods. Superfoods and sirtfoods are essentially within the same family. Sirtfoods may also be considered as superfoods. Both have common functions within the body and provide greater advantages than the typical diet. The sirtfoods are fantastic for low inflammation, promoting metabolism, loss of weight, immunity, and stable aging.

So, what kinds of foods do this new diet include? Here are a few: green tea, dark chocolate (over 85 percent cocoa), turmeric, kale, blueberries, parsley, capers, citrus fruit, apples, red wine, buckwheat, celery, chili, coffee, extra virgin olive oil, Medjool dates, red chicory, red onion, arugula, strawberries, and walnuts. The goal is not to consume a diet made entirely of such items but to integrate them as much as you can into your meals. For starters, it would be nice to have a smoothie composed of kale, blueberries, strawberries, and a splash of turmeric. This may also be a good choice for all the java lovers out there because this is one diet that really promotes the joe morning cup. These products are filled with polyphenols that are antioxidants that strengthen your skin and core.

The Sirtfood Diet is broken down into two stages. The first process, which lasts three days, allows you to restrict your daily calorie intake by consuming three green juices and one sirtfood-rich meal a day to 1000 calories a day. (You raise your meal count from days 4 to 7 to two meals and two green juices a day) The second process, the "maintenance" process, lasts 14 days and allows you to consume three sirtuin-rich meals and one green juice a day.

This book is a tool to help you live out this lifestyle to the fullest. You will find not only an evidence-based review, but potential health benefits are listed out. There are also recipes to help you get a jump start on your Sirtfood Diet! This lifestyle diet will allow you to live healthy all while enjoying your favorites. With that knowledge, the next time you are at your local grocery store, fill your cart full of Two-Buck Chuck and Hershey's Kisses. Enjoy your life and take control of your health!

Medical authorities caution that this diet may not measure up to the expectations. If you have pre-existing conditions, please consult your doctor before starting this diet.

WHAT IS THE SIRTFOOD DIET?

The Sirtfood Diet was created by two celebrity nutritionists working with a private gym in the UK. They market the diet as a radical modern lifestyle and wellness program that works by flipping the "skinny switch" on. This is done by focusing on sirtuin research (SIRTs), seven proteins within the body that have shown evidence of having control over several functions including: metabolism, inflammation, and lifespan. Some compounds from natural plants increase the body's protein, and the foods it contains are referred to as 'sirt foods.'

The science behind the diet is all about these proteins and finding them in food, otherwise known as Sirtfoods. Sirtfoods a group of newly discovered daily plant foods, high in a chemical compound known as sirtuin activators. These activators are a type of protein that flips on the body pathways of the so-called 'skinny gene.' Additionally, these pathways are the same ones stimulated more frequently through fasting and exercise. Both result in helping the body lose weight, raise muscle mass, and improve a healthy lifestyle.

Sirtfood Diet's compilation of "The Best 20 Sirtfoods" includes:

- Kale
- Red wine
- Strawberries
- Onions
- Soy
- Parsley
- Extra virgin olive oil
- Dark chocolate (85% cocoa)
- Matcha green tea
- Buckwheat
- Turmeric
- Walnuts
- Arugula (rocket)
- Bird's eye chili
- Lovage
- Medjool dates
- Red chicory

- Blueberries
- Capers
- Coffee

Goggins and Matten emphasis that adopting the Sirtfood diet can result in rapid weight loss, thus retaining muscle mass and shielding you from chronic disease. Upon finishing the program, you are encouraged to resume your regular diet with sirt products and the popular green juice of the diet. Fasting diets have been the main craze over the last couple of years, especially something like the 5:2 plan that became the-diet-to-do in 2015. But the Sirtfood plan is meant to imitate a fasting diet's weight loss effects – without sacrificing on health, fitness, muscle mass or food quality. This is thanks to new studies into this specific food group.

While being an effective weight loss program, Goggins and Matten stress that it is not just a diet plan but a health and wellness regime. The miraculous argument is that if you observe the sirtfood diet closely, you can lose 7 pounds in 7 days. Do not worry-despite dramatic lies, I am not a huge fan of fad diets. The framework is fascinating, and the underlying nutritional objective is something that I consider to be rather achievable, so listen to us! If I have not had your focus yet, there is going to be cookies and champagne.

In the first week, you need to adhere to a specific eating plan. Week one relies on you to have a little commitment. It sounds a little restricting and 'cleanse-like initially,' but it does get better. Every day you will want to reach for about 1,000 calories with three glasses of green juice and one lunch that is rich in sirt foods. In time, you will begin to increase your calorie intake to 1,500 calories, this happens in the second week and includes two green juices and two sirt-rich meals. Despite watching your daily intake of calories, the sirtfood diet does not have any clear rhyme or explanation, which is why I like it so much! The idea is to simply include as many sirt foods as possible in your diet to activate the sirtuins. This will keep our cells vibrant and healthy pushing us towards our goals!

Generally, I think the addition of more vitamins and mineral-rich whole grains in the diet and focus on greens is a smart solution. In addition, the long-term plan involves three sirtfood-rich meals a day, along with green tea. You should continue to see gradual weight loss at a safe pace throughout the following weeks post-introduction

Goggins and Matten make ambitious promises in claiming that the diet will induce super-charge weight loss, turn the "skinny gene" on and avoid disease. However, they face a problem. There is little much evidence to support their claim. To date, there is no convincing evidence that the Sirtfood Diet has a more beneficial effect on weight loss than any other diet limited by calories. While many of those foods have medicinal properties, no long-term human trials have been performed to establish if consuming a diet abundant in sirt foods has any measurable health benefits. Nevertheless, a pilot study was carried out by the founders, involving 39 participants from their fitness center. You can find this study published in the Sirtfood Diet journal. However, results of this study do not appear to have been published elsewhere.

Participants adopted the plan for a week and were required to walk every day. Participants weighed a total of 7 pounds (3.2 kg) less at the end of the week and retained or even added muscle mass. Those results, though, are hardly unexpected. Limiting your calorie consumption to 1,000 calories and concurrently exercising would almost certainly induce weight loss. Regardless, this kind of accelerated weight reduction is neither real nor long-lasting. As a result, this research did not track participants after the first week to see whether they gained some of the weight back, as it usually occurs. When the body becomes sugar-deprived, it utilizes its emergency nutrition reserves or glycogen. Each glycogen molecule requires 3–4 water molecules for storage. When your body uses glycogen, that water also gets rid of it. It is classified as "weight in mud." About one-third of the weight reduction occurs from fat during the first week of severe calorie restriction, while the remaining two-thirds come from skin, food, and glycogen. Your body must replenish its glycogen reserves if the calorie consumption rises, thus the weight comes right back. Unfortunately, in addition, this kind of calorie reduction will even cause the body to reduce its metabolic rate. Resulting in you consuming far less energy-efficient calories each day.

As far as disease prevention is concerned, it is certain that three weeks is not long enough to have any meaningful long-term effects. On the other side, it might be a smart decision to introduce sirtfood to your daily diet for the long term. However, you may as well miss the detox portion and start in sirtfoods now.

The diet is split into two phases; the initial period lasts one week and includes a three-day reduction in calories to 1000 kcal, intake in three sirtfood green juices and one meal rich in sirt foods. The juices contain spinach, celery, rocket, parsley, lemon, and green tea. Meals contain turkey escalope with buckwheat noodles, basil, capers and parsley, chicken and kale curry, and prawn stir-fry. Your calorie intakes for days four through seven are increased to 1500kcal, consisting of two sirtfood green juices and two sirtfood-rich meals a day. You must also be consuming water consistently, with the recommended quantities meeting the existing average requirements during step one.

The second period is regarded as the 14-day maintenance process, where there is a slow weight loss. Goggins and Matten believe that this period is practical and a safe way to lose weight. Focusing on weight reduction, though, is not what the diet is about – it is about consuming the best food that nature must bring. They suggest three healthy sirtfood-rich meals a day together with one sirtfood-green juice in the long term.

DIETITIAN EMER DELANEY SAYS:

'This is not a lifestyle I would prescribe to someone at first glance. It is incredibly challenging to strive for 1000kcal for three consecutive days, so I assume that most people will not be able to do this. Looking at the food page, you will see that they are the sort of things that sometimes occur on a 'good food chart,' but as part of a more balanced diet, it will be easier to promote them. Occasionally enjoying a glass of red wine or a tiny quantity of candy would do us no good-I would not suggest it every day. We will consume a mixture of numerous fruits and vegetables and not all those on the list as well.

'People may have undergone a seven-pound weight drop on the scales in terms of weight reduction and improving metabolism, but in my opinion, it would be air. It takes time to burn and lose fat, so this weight loss is extremely unlikely to be a loss of fat. I should be cautious of any diet that promotes quick and rapid weight loss because that is obviously not possible and is more than a fluid loss. They should recover their weight as people adjust to their normal eating habits. Slow and steady weight loss is the key, and for that, we need to limit calories and increase our levels of activity. The best way to lose weight is to consume healthy daily meals made up of low GI

ingredients, lean protein, fruit, and vegetables, and stay well hydrated.'

PHASES OF THE SIRTFOOD DIET

After the three weeks going through the two phases of the Sirtfood Diet, you can continue to "sirtify" your diet by including as many sirt foods as possible into your meals. The basic recipes for these two phases can be found in the book *The Sirtfood Diet*. There are many sirt foods used in the meals, but there are additional foods listed in the "Top 20 Sirt Foods." Most sirtfoods and ingredients are easy to find. There are three signature foods during the two phases — matcha green tea powder, lovage, and buckwheat — which unlike many of the sirt foods can be costly or hard to find.

A large part of the diet is its green juice, which you will consume between one to three times a day. A juicer a kitchen scale will be needed, as the ingredients are listed by weight. Blenders will not work in gaining the consistency that you need. The recipe is below:

SIRTFOOD GREEN JUICE

- 75 grams (2.5 oz) kale
- 30 grams (1 oz) arugula (rocket)
- five grams parsley
- two celery sticks
- one cm (0.5 in) ginger
- ½ of a green apple
- ½ of a lemon
- ½ of a teaspoon matcha green tea

Juice all ingredients, *except green tea powder and lemon*, and pour into a glass. Squeeze the lemon by hand, then mix the lemon juice and green tea powder into the juice. Enjoy!

PHASE ONE

The first phase lasts for seven days, with calorie restriction and lots of green juice involved. It is meant to boost your weight loss and claims to help you lose 7 pounds (3.2 kg) in seven days. Intake of calories during the first three days of phase one is limited to 1,000 calories. You drink three green drinks, plus one dish, every day. You will select from recipes in the book every day, many of which include sirtfood as a big part of the meal.

Examples are miso-glazed tofu, the omelet sirtfood, or the buckwheat stir-fry shrimp. On days four through seven of Phase One, your calorie consumption is raised to 1,500 per day. This involves two green juices a day and two more sirt-rich meals that can be picked from the book.

PHASE TWO

Phase two takes two weeks to complete. You should continue to lose weight steadily during this "maintenance" phase. This phase has no specific calorie limit. Instead, you eat three sirt-fed meals and one green juice a day. The meals are again selected from the recipes found in the book.

AFTER THE DIET

The two stages can be replicated as much as you want for more weight reduction. However, after completing the phases, you are encouraged to continue "sirtifying" your diet by regularly incorporating sirt foods into your meals. Sirtfood Diet books are numerous, and there is an abundance of sirtfood recipes. Sirt foods can also be used as a snack in your diet or in your meals. You are also advised to drink the green juice every day.

IS SIRTFOODS THE NEW SUPERFOODS?

There is no denying how good sirt foods are. They also have strong nutrient content and are made of good plant compounds. In fact, reports have linked the health benefits of many of the sirt food choices. Eating moderate amounts of dark chocolate with a high content of cacao, for example, can reduce the risk of heart disease and help fight inflammation. Drinking green tea can lower the risk of stroke and diabetes and reduce blood pressure. Turmeric has anti-inflammatory properties that generally have beneficial effects on the body and can protect against chronic inflammatory diseases. Most sirtfoods have demonstrated health benefits in humans.

Evidence on the health benefits shows that increasing the levels of sirtuin protein is the primary benefit. Yet animal and cell line research have been showing exciting results. For example, researchers have shown that higher levels of some sirtuin proteins contribute to longer lifetimes for leaves, worms, and mice. A rise in sirtuin levels resulted in a fat drop in one mice sample. Some evidence suggests sirtuins may also play a role in reducing inflammation, inhibiting tumor development, and slowing heart disease and

Alzheimer's development. While studies have shown positive results in mice and human cell lines, no human studies have examined the effects of increasing sirtuin levels. Therefore, it is unknown whether increased levels of sirtuin protein in the body will lead to a longer lifespan or a lower risk of human cancer. Current research is underway to develop compounds that are effective at increasing sirtuin levels in the body. This allows human studies to start examining the effects of sirtuins on human health. Until then, the effects of increased sirtuin levels cannot be determined.

Is It Healthy And Sustainable?

Sirtfoods are nearly all healthy choices and can even have health benefits because of their antioxidant or anti-inflammatory properties. But consuming just a handful of especially nutritious foods cannot fulfill all the nutritional needs of the body. The diet is restrictive and does not provide any simple or special health benefits over any other diet. Additionally, consuming just 1,000 calories is not usually advised without a doctor's supervision. For many people, even eating 1,500 calories per day is overly restrictive.

In addition, the diet requires up to three green juices per day. Though juices can be a good source of vitamins and minerals, they are also a source of sugar and have almost none of the nutritious fibers that whole fruits and vegetables do. All-day sipping on juice is a bad idea for both your blood sugar and your teeth. Not to mention, as the diet is so restricted in calories and food options, nutrients, vitamins, and minerals are more than likely insufficient, particularly during the first step. Due to low calories restrictions and limited food options, it is challenging to adhere to this diet for a full three weeks. Add to the initial high cost of purchasing a juicer, a book and other unusual, pricey ingredients and the time taken to prepare other foods and juices, many people cannot afford and cannot maintain this diet.

Safety and Side Effects

Although low calories and nutrients are included in the first step of the diet, there are no concerns for healthy adults, despite the limited diet. However, for someone with diabetes, limiting calories and mostly drinking juice for the first few days of the diet may cause dangerous changes in blood sugar levels. Likewise, even a healthy individual can encounter certain side effects — primarily hunger. Eating just 1,000–1,500 calories per day will leave just about anyone feeling hungry, especially if much of what you are eating is juice that is low in fiber, a nutrient that helps you stay full. During phase one, due to the calorie restriction, you might experience other side effects such as fatigue, lightheadedness, and irritability. Serious health effects are impossible for a healthy person if the plan is adopted for a mere three weeks. Sirtfood Diet is rich in nutritious foods, but not perfect in dietary habits.

Its theory and health claims are based on great scientific extrapolations. While adding some sirt food to your diet and maybe promising some health benefits is not a bad thing, the diet itself looks like a different fad.

Save time and then save money to make long-term, balanced lifestyle improvements.

MAINTAIN THE HEALTHY WEIGHT

WITH 52% OF AMERICANS ADMITTING THAT THEY DISCOVER IT SIMPLER TO DO THEIR TAXES THAN TO COMPREHEND HOW TO EAT A HEALTHY DIET, IT IS CRUCIAL TO INTRODUCE A KIND OF EATING THAT BECOMES A LIFESTYLE RATHER THAN A ONE-OFF CRASH DIET. FOR A FEW OF US, IT MAY NOT BE THAT TOUGH TO DROP WEIGHT OR RETAIN A HEALTHY WEIGHT; HOWEVER, THE SIRTFOOD DIET PLAN CAN ASSIST THOSE WHO ARE STRUGGLING. WHAT ABOUT INTEGRATING THE SIRTFOOD DIET PLAN WITH A WORKOUT, IS IT A GOOD IDEA TO PREVENT EXERCISE ENTIRELY OR PRESENT IT WHEN YOU HAVE BEGUN THE DIET PLAN?

THE SIRT DIET PRINCIPLES

With an estimated 650 million obese adults globally, it is essential to find healthy eating and exercise routines that are achievable. Do not deny you of whatever you delight in, and do not require strenuous workouts every day of the week. The Sirtfood diet allows you to accomplish this. The concept is that foods will activate the 'skinny gene' pathways, which are typically activated by fasting and exercise. The bright side is that some foods and beverages, consisting of dark chocolate and red wine, consists of chemicals called polyphenols that trigger the genes that imitate the results of exercise and fasting.

EXERCISE DURING THE FIRST FEW WEEKS

During the first two weeks of the diet plan, where your calorie intake is minimized, it would be sensible to stop or lower workout while your body adjusts to fewer calories. Understand and listen to your body. Do not exercise if you are exhausted or have less strength than normal. Instead, ensure that you stay focused on the principles that make up a healthy lifestyle such as consisting of sufficient everyday levels of fiber, protein and fruit and veggies.

BECOMING A LIFESTYLE

When you do exercise, it is important to take in protein, preferably an hour after your workout. Protein repair work muscles after a workout lower pain and can aid healing. There are various types of sauces that provide this protein: the sirt chili con carne or the turmeric chicken and the kale salad. Both are suitable for after exercise consumptions. If you desire something lighter, you can try the sirt blueberry healthy smoothie and include some protein powder for added advantage.

The Sirtfood Diet is a fantastic way to change your eating practices, reduce weight and feel healthier. The preliminary few weeks may challenge you, but it is necessary to examine which foods are best to consume and which scrumptious recipes match you. Be kind to yourself in the first couple of weeks while your body adapts and take exercise easy if you select to do it at all. If you are already somebody who does extreme or moderate exercise, then it might be that you can continue as typical or manage your physical fitness in accordance with the change in diet. Like any diet plan and workout changes, it is important to only push yourself as far as your body allows.

PERSONAL EXPERIENCE: 14-DAY SAMPLE MEAL PLAN

Week One:

DAY 1/ MONDAY (3 JUICES, 1 MEAL).

Once I learned how to manage my new juicer and do some healthy kick-start shopping, I was all set to go. I was not confident about the first three days going through the sirtfood diet with only three green juices and one lunch. In truth, however, I was happily stunned. The juices were drinkable, and bizarrely, I did not feel hungry throughout the day up until about 5 pm (which was just an hour prior to dinner, so entirely manageable). I spaced the juices out, and then I had one at 7:30 am (our regular breakfast time), one at 11:00 am, one at 2:30 pm and then dinner at 6 pm. Supper was this tasty, King Prawn stir fry with buckwheat noodles. You will find this recipe in the back of this book. The genuine emphasis of the day was the two squares of Lindt 85% chocolate I was permitted after supper. I waited until my kids remained in bed, and I had completed work for the day. Then, I allowed myself this treat, and it was fantastic. Prior to heading off to bed, I comprised my three juices for the next day for more efficiency.

DAY 2/ TUESDAY (3 JUICES, 1 MEAL).

Feeling smug that I had completed Monday so well and had all my juices all set to go, Tuesday was something of a shocker. The juice, which I had been rather pleased drinking on Monday, tasted vile – enough so that it made me gag! I am not sure what failed here. I have a couple of theories: (1) possibly making it the night prior to making the juices were less fresh, (2) possibly the kale I used in batch 2 of the juices was a bit past its best, (3) maybe my body had all of a sudden altered its mind and rejected the juice? Still uncertain what the reasons were, but by juice three on Tuesday, I simply could not drink it— All-day! All-day! – not even holding it up to my nose. I had some snacks leaving the rest of the juice 3 dropped the sink. Two selections for dinner are accessible daily: one meat/fish and one veggie/vegan: kale and red onion dhal. After all of this, a wonderful decadent treat of 2 Lindt squares. Following my green juice fiasco, I was determined that I would not pre-make my juices the night before but rather keep it new every week on Wednesday. My Tesco man got here with a fresh batch of kale, so the old, nasty kale went in the bin.

DAY 3/ WEDNESDAY (3 JUICES, 1 MEAL).

On Wednesday, I made a few changes to the juice. I upped the apple— a whole apple, not half as per the recipe. Then I reduced the celery marginally, this was the big scent that gagged me. The celery reduced from 2 to 1 ring. However, just like Monday and Tuesday, I included the water. It was great! Although not the most delicious thing I have ever tainted in my career, but it was drinkable (unlike the poor Tuesday sample that was not!).

A thought was niggling in my brain, as the diet plan started. The components of Sirtfood green juice all looked like pretty fabulous salad active ingredients. Is it going to work? Okay, I thought it worth a try! I used the ingredients instead of juice 2 to make an easy salad. Out of lemon juice and ginger, I made a dressing with a little extra virgin olive oil. I mixed it and then included the apple, celery, and parsley, plus several walnuts. Walnuts and other virgin olive oil are both Sirtfoods, but I did not feel guilty to add them... and yeah, it made a lovely salad! The salad was huge. I could not even finish it all, but it smelt amazing. Clearly, this one had to be even better compared to the juice water!!

Wednesday's supper was another triumph: aromatic chicken with kale, buckwheat, and salsa. It was delicious and extremely simple to do. That salsa though... I might have consumed an entire bucket of that – so great! My only grievance would be that it used every pot and pan in the home (OKAY I exaggerate. It used five. Yet this is more than I normally would use – I am one pot of a woman, but often two and rarely five, unless it is like Christmas or something and then... You see my Holiday Turkey Recipe Tray bake?). I think that anyone who writes the Sirtfood dishes must have someone to wash for him. (The quick check of the book shows that it is a chef named Mark McCulloch, so he probably has a whole army of helpers to wash up!).

And after that, there was the chocolate again. You need to envision me at about 9pm, on the sofa, checking out a book, eating chocolate, and drinking chamomile tea. I am so extremely happy. It is a very, great method to end the day!

DAY 4/ THURSDAY (2 JUICES, 2 MEALS).

On Day 4, it is all about modifications, and you have enabled two proper meals and two green juices. This provided me a little an issue regarding when to have the first meal. I made the Sirt muesli, which is more of a breakfast thing really, but I wished to spread the meals out a bit, so I chose to have the muesli at 11 am and the juices at 7:30 am and 2:30 pm. I do think my wonderful Juicer was one of the things that made the green juice so bearable. In fact, I enjoy it and will certainly make more juices once I finish the Sirtfood Diet (although I might have a break for some time from the kale and celery!). The Sirt muesli was FAB and one of my weeks one is two utter highlights (the other is Saturday's snack! See below). It was so easy to make, honestly. You can do loads in one go. Plus, it tastes amazing! Furthermore, the volume you are allowed is immense-I could not consume everything!

For supper, I went with the vegan alternative of Tuscan bean stew. There is a salmon alternative, if you prefer, which also sounds great. The stew was very good, but it was the third meal in a row eaten with sweet weed. It would have been perfect if something else had been served as I was overflowing with sweet weed at this stage. Buckwheat is fine, but not every day, the same goes for kale and celery. I understand the Sirtfood Diet attempts to pack in as much of the top 20 Sirtfoods as possible into each meal; however, it does make for a bit too much sameness. I do like kale/celery/buckwheat etc. But for breakfast lunch and supper every day for a week – not so much!

Here are the important things now. There is no longer any reference after Wednesday of the Chocolate, which I believe was a mistake! (extremely naughty) I have chosen to go on with the 85% Lindt. Oh well... It is Sirtfood! It is Sirtfood!

DAY 5/ FRIDAY (2 JUICES, 2 MEALS).

Friday began with a green juice, just like all my other days, but it was a school sport and a lunch day. This made for a very difficult time eating or preparing my sirtfoods. One I got home, I chose to make the juices and eat a gloriously portable strawberry buckwheat tabbouleh while going out for a picnic. It was so good, so much more than a sandwich. The Sirtfood Diet works fantastically around a genuine life.

Dinner was miso marinated baked cod and, once again, tasty but with more kale and buckwheat. My family was a bit cross about having to consume buckwheat once again. And yes. There was more chocolate. I am sorry. I could not help myself!

DAY 6/ SATURDAY (2 JUICES, 2 MEALS).

Today the kids and my other half were home, so I had juice for breakfast and after that the sirtfood meals for lunch and dinner. Lunch was the Sirtfood Super Salad, a tasty mix of rocket, chicory, avocado, walnuts, capers, and a whole host of other sirtfoods. The protein portion of the salad has four choices: lentils, salmon fried, chicken or tuna— I selected the chicken, but I would have been very pleased with any of these. I had chicken and salad on my own, and my husband and children had sandwiches with it. I put all the different elements of the salad on the table in small bowls to help all of them (so my kids were pleased not having to eat around what they did not like).

The real emphasis of the day was supper: chargrilled beef with red wine gravy and herb roasted potatoes. All I can say is it was yum yummy! It was another 'every pan in the home' meal and did involve yet more kale! That red wine gravy was simply remarkable—I will absolutely be making that once again. Although the diet is hailed as red wine and chocolate, the wine is strictly excluded at week one (afterward, you can get 2-3 glasses a week if you like). I have been strong and stayed driven. The irony was that there was red wine in the sauce. But it was a tough one. Good steak in my universe requires a great red wine! My other half had with him a bottle of Cabernet Sauvignon, which went so well. And I had chocolate again, of course!

DAY 7/ SUNDAY (2 JUICES, 2 MEALS).

Sunday was a truly hectic day with lots going on in the early morning, and I knew lunch would be late. The idea of getting through up until 2pm on juice alone was not appealing. So… I cheated. Only slightly by having a bowl of that scrumptious Sirt muesli instead. Oh my, those things are soooo excellent!

Lunch was a marvelous bacon sirtfood omelet. You can officially put the bacon in the omelet, but instead, I got mine on the side… Well, I might have had three bacon pieces... but I was very hectic early in the morning.

I do not live with big fans of red onions or tomatoes, I made them a "normal" salad and served with crusty white bread for them and my mother. I just enjoyed the chicken and red onion salad for them. I changed the salad a little by using some capers and lemon juice rather than bright, white vinegar.

SIRTFOOD DIET WEEK 1: REFLECTIONS AND SUGGESTIONS

TOO MUCH FOOD/ PORTION SIZES/ RANDOM QUANTITIES

The portion sizes of the sirtfood diet are my greatest issue and tended to ruin the focus of a diet schedule. I would rather consume two smaller meals a day than one big one. I could not completely eat. In some instances, they were not super-sized servings, just percentages–like crazy amounts of kale with steak and two cherry tomatoes in a salsa (if you do it for 4). I urge you to make a sound judgment and to do as much as you believe fair if the book suggests unhealthy food when you do the sirtfood diet. In their second book, the authors state that if you feel complete, you should stop eating and not force yourself to end up with a portion that is too great.

ABSENCE OF VARIETY

In week one, I was fed up with kale, celery, and buckwheat 100%. Too much of an outstanding thing can surely be avoided!! It would be perfect if the food policy had a little more variety. I recommend you avoid too much variety if you plan to blend and match.

WEIGHT-LOSS AND OTHER BENEFITS

I lost 5lb in the very first three days!! With how much I was drinking, I am not sure it is was from flushing out water weight. The unique thing about this diet plan is that it is supposed to help you gain muscle as well as lose weight. I do not have expensive scales that inform me such things. Based on the book, I cannot say why people normally put a little weight into muscle and lose weight in fat, so it is completely possible that I gained muscle in place and lost more fat.

For me, the diet was so much more than about losing weight. I was intrigued to see if I could take advantage of any of the other claims ... and the response is yes! I absolutely feel healthier; I have been sleeping better, I feel more energetic and positive, more alert (and no it's not due to the fact that of the coffee – I said goodbye to coffee on most days) and bizarrely I have felt less hungry! I have also been drinking more water, and now I understand that often when I feel starving, I am most likely thirsty ... or just tired!

SIRTFOOD DIET WEEK 2 SAMPLE

DAY 8 MONDAY

It was so good to have three meals a day back!! The juice in the diet was good and helped me lose 6 lbs., but the much frustrating part of the diet now is the "maintenance" phase! You are given three balanced sirtfood meals a day plus one or two small meals. Today started with a sirtfood smoothie, which was okay, however, not as great as the sirtfood muesli. It was a little frustrating that after seven days off breakfast, the very first breakfast you are permitted is in liquid form!

Lunch was far more exciting: I had another chicken sirtfood super salad, which was just as great as it was on Saturday. I had baked an extra chicken breast on Sunday supper time, so this salad took simple minutes to throw together. Dinner required to be flexible as my husband was getting back late, so I chose the vegetable alternative of Tuscan bean stew again, which was extremely easy to make and tasted terrific.

On Monday night, I did my weekly store run – it was a little more pricey than my normal grocery trip. However, not by much and it was simple to do, as I had already got all the complicated things in before I began the diet. I primarily stayed with the strategy; however, I switched in a few meals from The Sirtfood Diet Recipe Book. I was impressed at simply how household-friendly the book is. There are lots of household favorites such as spaghetti Bolognese, fajitas, chicken korma and beef bourguignon. In truth, by the time I had finished, I had a list that was far too long of all the meals I wished to attempt!

And yes, I did maintain my little Lindt 85% chocolate routine – practically all week in fact!

DAY 9 TUESDAY

Breakfast was the fantastic sirtfood muesli again, which was as nice as it had constantly been. This really is a fabulous method to begin the day and fills me up remarkably. I do not feel hungry once again while waiting for lunchtime. Tuesday was my daughter's school trip day, so I went as one of my parent helpers. I wanted something that served well as a packed lunch to take with me. Luckily, the lunch arranged for Tuesday was whole meal pittas. Perfect for a jam-packed lunch. Nevertheless, I have a strong hostility towards soaking sandwiches, so I packed anything that I needed and made them at lunch rather than making the pittas in the morning. It was much for the fun of my child's schoolmates!

After a long day, it was easy to throw together the evening meal-a tasty butternut squash and toast. I was a little worried that with the butternut squash and the dates, it would be too sweet. However, in fact, it was ok, and the sweet taste worked so well with the cinnamon. I would truly like to try this again but with lamb in it too, as I can think of the cinnamon and dates would go so effectively with lamb. (*I did ultimately remake this tagine with lamb, and it was incredible!!*) The tagine was served with yet more buckwheat, however really by this point, I was starting to get a taste for the buckwheat! I believe it had become an acquired taste. Now that I am accustomed to it, I am really enjoying it. Even the kids did not grumble this time!

DAY 10 WEDNESDAY

For breakfast, I had Greek yogurt with combined berries, chocolate, and walnuts – a rather decadent reward for breakfast and much better than Monday's shake. Way better than the green juices! I added a couple of coconut flakes for extra scrumptiousness. Lunch would once again be the sirtfood super salad, but I wanted to have pittas again because of some active ingredients I had leftover. I believe one method this diet might be enhanced by is identifying that you may have some leftover components from the previous day and reusing them the next day.

The children and I had a wonderful time after school creating these fun sirtfood bites. You should have 1 to 2 a day. On Wednesday, I normally go for a run with my running group, so a couple of sirtfood bites were simply ideal for giving me the energy for a 4.5-mile run. Ok, so it was, in fact, 4 sirtfood bites that I consumed.

Wednesday's dinner was a delicious chili con carne, that was just right for a day that we all had to eat at different times. I made chilies for children and then heated them up for my other half and me later. The children had it with white rice, while the hubby and I had the buckwheat was ours. The chili was quite a basic recipe, but it had plenty of chilies, red wine, turmeric, and cocoa. It smelled great, but not as good as my chili beef. Next time I make the chili beef, I hope I can try adding some chocolate, red wine, and turmeric to it!

DAY 11 THURSDAY

Thursday's breakfast was expected to be spiced scrambled eggs; however, the concept of cooking and eating scrambled eggs at 7:30 on a hectic school morning just was not appealing. So, I made the terrific sirtfood muesli instead. To shake things up, I added some blueberries and raspberries to the mix.

Lunch was expected to be the strawberry buckwheat tabbouleh once again; however, I decided that I would rather fancy having a go at something else, so instead, I made this rather incredible potato salad to go with rainbow trout and watercress, a dish from The Sirtfood Recipe Book. I also added in a handful of the rocket for additional sirtfood goodness. This one was among the stand apart meals of the week and extremely simple to assemble. You only roast a couple of new potatoes and then dress the hot pads in a quick mix of capers, red onions, lemon juice, extra virgin olive oil, celery, and parsley. Include a cooked all-packed fillet of smoked trout and a selection of watercresses. I could not get enough of this!

I was feeling slightly peckish at about 4pm, and sadly we had polished off all the srtfood bites the day before. I did not have time to make anymore, so rather, I had a handful of walnuts and a date. I figured because they were both sirtfoods and active ingredients in the sirtfood bites, they would make an excellent alternative. It would be nice to have a few tips for fast and simple treats in the books, though. There are no guidelines for fast and simple remedies, but the recipe book does have several snack recipes.

Dinner was a thing I was looking forward to, because I started the diet first: Bombay potatoes, chicken, and kale curry. I adapted the recipe slightly with chicken thighs rather than breast fillets but kept the same recipe generally otherwise. It was a great curry, but by no means, my favorite meal of the week and the Bombay potatoes were a bit boring – more like yellow roasted potatoes than Bombay potatoes!

DAY 12 FRIDAY

Despite putting on a pound, I have still been reaping the rewards of a healthy diet. I am still feeling very much 'bright-eyed and bushy-tailed' and continue to sleep incredibly well. Friday's breakfast was a re-run of Wednesdays, with Greek Yogurt, fresh fruit, cacao nibs, walnuts, and coconut flakes. Completely scrumptious and quickly kept me going up until lunch. I should have had the sirtfood smoothie, but I decided the yogurt and fruit option would be much nicer, and it was!

For lunch, I decided to have the sirtfood super salad, rather than the Walldorf salad on the strategy. I am delighting in the fact that you can match and mix and swap in various things, depending upon what you wish. This time I selected to have some leftover feta cheese instead of chicken in my salad. With no 'main' option, I had some of Wednesday's leftover pittas. I understood it would go remarkably well with the other active ingredients, especially the rocket, avocado and walnuts-- and it did! I will be having this variation rather. I, in fact, preferred it to the chicken choice.

I did attempt to keep the journal as complimentary as possible for the three weeks of the sirtfood diet; however, it was impossible to discover three weeks with definitely nothing scheduled and we had actually had this Friday's earmarked as a 'date night' for months. I expect I might have canceled it; however, my partner and I have date nights so infrequently that, well, I did not wish to! We chose to go ahead and go out to a dining establishment as we had originally planned.

This did provide me a bit of an issue sirtfood-wise. There are no directions for what to do at a restaurant in the book. Certainly, I could not call up the dining establishment and ask them to make buckwheat pasta with smoked salmon, chili, and rocket, as per the strategy! I chose just to go with little portions and just one glass of white wine. We went to a lovely Thai dining establishment-- which was fantastic as I knew I would get at least a couple of sirtfoods, such as chili, shallots, spices, herbs and nuts, and all essential glass of white wine. I likewise had a coffee later rather than pudding. I can inform you, after 12 days of abstaining, that glass of wine tasted excellent indeed!

DAY 13 SATURDAY

As I was running a 10k on Saturday morning, I realized that I wanted some essential food— and I had not had the time to make the pancakes that were on the schedule. I have been looking at my buckwheat flakes and questioning if they might make a great porridge all week, so I decided Saturday would be a great day to provide it a go. The dates and the cocoa I made were a combination of buckwheat flakes. I added a combination of walnuts and berries to complete it. If I can claim that and good for my sprint, not a poor coffee substitute, it seemed to do the trick, I had gas! Then 5 minutes shaved my old PB!!

Lunch was expected to be tofu and shitake mushroom soup, which sounded great to me, but I could not imagine anybody else in my family would be particularly delighted with it, so I swapped in another dish from the Sirtfood Diet Recipe Book of grilled sausages with herby scrambled eggs. I somewhat adjusted the dish by adding in some turmeric and chili to the eggs to make them additional sirtfoodie!! My kids were not convinced and declined to try the eggs, rather plumping for toast and baked beans to opt for their sausages. My hubby had all the above!

Saturday night was even more difficult to manage than Friday night. We had been invited round to a buddy's home for a murder mystery celebration. Where the menu is a seafood dish with poisoning, a mashed potato, and then a dessert option: pavlova or banoffee pie— both good, yet hardly a sirt food in sight. Now clearly you cannot go to someone's house for supper and then call them up and ask for the menu to consist of lots of sirtfoods. Again, neither of the books offers any advice for this situation! I decided to choose roughly the very same plan as the night prior to small portions and my remaining two glasses of white wine for the week! I almost managed to stay with my strategy; however, it was really hard-- specifically when the cheese course came out! I was rather unfortunate not to be able to try either of the two whiskeys that evening

DAY 14 SUNDAY

I had a bit more time on Sunday morning, So I chose to make pancakes sirtfood, which was supposed to be the breakfast of Saturday. My only grievance would be that the dish called for one tablespoon of double cream, and there were no other dishes that called for double cream in the next couple of days, suggesting the cream would have been squandered. If it had not been for the reality, my kids and other half assured to help me polish it off!

For Sunday lunch, we had pittas again with more feta cheese, lemon, and coriander humus this time, very scrumptious. The kids were able to choose what they could put into their pittas. We had pizzas dinner on Saturday night. Like the biscuits, buckwheat flour was used in pizzas. The tomato sauce often contains red onion for additional sirtfood. There are numerous ideas for garnishes; however, I chose goats cheese, rocket, and chili for me and my spouse. I let the kids select what they wished to have, and they opted for cheddar cheese, mushrooms, peppers, and oregano. But we all had a good time making and eating the pizzas and it was a lovely thing to do as a household on a Sunday afternoon. A beautiful end to week 2 of the Sirtfood Diet.

SIRTFOOD DIET WEEK 2: REFLECTIONS AND SUGGESTIONS

A DIET FOR FOODIES

Week One was quite great, however in Week two the dishes got even better. Highlights have included, the fantastic sirtfood chili, the terrific potato salad, those chocolate-covered pancakes, and the terrific sirtfood pizzas-- and I have been expecting what I prepare to cook next week.

HEALTH BENEFITS

I have not really lost any weight this week. I put a pound on, which is a bit unfortunate-- but barely surprising considering that today featured a journey to a dining establishment and a supper party! But I have continued to experience all the other advantages of the Sirtfood Diet that I experienced in the very first week-- more so in truth now I am eating appropriately. I am feeling incredibly perky, extremely positive, and alert. I am likewise still sleeping like the proverbial infant. However, I think I should not be shocked because I am feeding my body great deals of extremely healthy foods, filled with minerals and vitamins, and not eating any junk/processed food/ improved carbs or sugar. I think possibly there is a lot to be said for the old saying: you are what you eat!

PORTION SIZES

One of my gripes last week was the part sizes appeared massive. I have not found that at all this week.

RANGE AND LEFTOVERS

Last week I got thoroughly fed up with kale, celery, and buckwheat. This week was a lot better-- a lot more variety! However, one problem I would make today exists was a lot of range that things did not get consumed. I had leftover pittas that would have gone to waste if I had not rearranged things to guarantee I utilized them up and leftover cream that fortunately my household finished up for me. It would likewise have actually been excellent if the meal plan had been written in a method that suggested you made extra of the dinners and utilized the leftovers up the next day for lunch, for that reason making my life much easier!

PARTIES AND DINING ESTABLISHMENTS

I tried to select a 3-week duration to do this diet plan where there were not going to be any social celebrations, but my life is so hectic. I quickly realized there was never going to be a 3-week duration where nothing occurred! One difficulty with this diet is it does not offer you much aid with how to handle dining establishments and dinner celebrations. It is a diet plan with a meal plan which says, 'consume this on this day.'

ARE SIRTFOODS THE NEW SUPERFOODS?

There is no denying that sirtfoods benefit you. They are frequently high in nutrients and complete healthy plant compounds. Moreover, research studies have associated many of the foods recommended on the Sirtfood Diet with health advantages. For example, consuming moderate amounts of dark chocolate with high cocoa content might decrease the danger of cardiovascular disease and assistance fight inflammation. Consuming green tea might decrease the risk of stroke and diabetes and help lower high blood pressure. Turmeric has anti-inflammatory properties that have advantageous impacts on the body in general and may even secure against chronic, inflammation-related illness. The bulk of sirtfoods have demonstrated health benefits in people.

Nevertheless, proof of the health advantages of increasing sirtuin protein levels is preliminary. Research in animals and cell lines has revealed exciting results. For instance, researchers have found that increased levels of certain sirtuin proteins cause longer lifespan in yeast, mice, and worms.

Throughout fasting or calorie limitation, sirtuin proteins inform the body to burn more fat for energy and improve insulin level of sensitivity. One study in mice discovered that increased sirtuin levels resulted in weight loss. Some evidence recommends that sirtuins may likewise play a role in minimizing swelling, hindering the advancement of growths, and slowing the development of cardiovascular disease and Alzheimer's.

While research studies in mice and human cell lines have revealed favorable results, there have been no human studies examining the effects of increasing sirtuin levels.

Whether increasing sirtuin protein levels in the body will lead to longer lifespan or a lower danger of cancer in humans is unknown. Research study is currently underway to develop substances efficient at increasing sirtuin levels in the body. By doing this, human research studies can begin to look at the effects of sirtuins on human health. Until then, it is not possible to identify the results of increased sirtuin levels. Sirtfoods are generally healthy foods. Extremely little is understood about how these foods affect sirtuin levels and human health.

IS IT EFFECTIVE?

The Sirtfood Diet's authors make bold statements that the diet will overburden weight loss, turn on the "lean gene," and avoid illness. However, there is no persuasive evidence that Sirtfood Diet has a more positive weight loss effect than any other limited calorie diet. Although many of these foods have healthful properties, there have not been any long-lasting human research studies to determine whether eating a diet rich in sirtfoods has any concrete health benefits.

Nonetheless, this sirtfood diet plan book reports the outcomes of a pilot study conducted by the authors and involving 39 individuals from their gym. For one week, the individuals followed the diet and worked out daily. At the end of the week, participants lost approximately 7 pounds (3.2 kg) and kept and/or gained muscle mass. Yet these outcomes are hardly surprising. Restricting your calorie intake to 1,000 calories and working out at the very same time will almost always trigger weight reduction. This study did not follow participants after the very first week to see if they regained any of the weight back, which is normally the case.

When your body is energy-deprived, it utilizes up its emergency energy stores, or glycogen, in addition to burning fat and muscle. Each particle of glycogen needs 3-- 4 particles of water to be kept. It gets rid of the water when your body is using glycogen. You may have heard this called "losing water weight". Only about one-third of weight loss comes from fat during the first week of extreme calorie stress, and the other two thirds from water, muscle, and glycogen. As your calories increase, the body renovates its glycogen reserves, and the weight recovers instantly. This type of calorie limitation can cause your body to decrease its metabolic rate, triggering you require even fewer calories per day for energy than before. It is most likely that this diet plan may assist you to lose a couple of pounds in the beginning, but it will likely come back as quickly once the diet plan is over.

This diet is also not compatible in the ability to see how it strengthens the body against illness. Three weeks is probably not long enough to have any measurable long-lasting effect. On another hand, it might be smart to add sirt food to your daily diet in the long run. Rather than using it as a diet, it can be used as a lifestyle change.

IS IT HEALTHY AND SUSTAINABLE?

Sirtfoods are nearly all healthy options and may even lead to some health benefits due to their anti-inflammatory or antioxidant residential or commercial properties. However, simply consuming a handful of particularly healthy foods can not satisfy all your body's dietary needs. Eating only 1,000 calories is normally not suggested without the supervision of a physician. Even consuming 1,500 calories per day is exceedingly limiting for many individuals.

The diet plan also includes drinking up to 3 green juices per day. Although juices can be a good source of minerals and vitamins, they are likewise a source of sugar and consist of nearly none of the healthy fiber that whole fruits and veggies do. Additionally, sipping on juice throughout the whole day is a bad concept for both your blood sugar and your teeth.

To make matters worse in the the diet plan being so minimal in calories and food choice, it is very much lacking in protein, vitamins, and minerals, specifically during the first stage. Due to the low-calorie levels and limiting food options, this diet plan may be challenging to adhere to for the whole three weeks. Add that to the high initial expenses of needing to buy a juicer, the book, and specific uncommon and costly components it can be too expensive for most. That does not include time expenses of preparing specific meals and juices. Altogether this diet plan ends up being unfeasible and unsustainable for many individuals.

HOW TO MAINTAIN THE HEALTHY WEIGHT GAINED WITH THE SIRT DIET

Too much weight is painful, and your wellbeing may also be affected. According to the Centers for Disease Control and Prevention (CDC), obesity levels have grown in the United States over the last few years. More than a third of American adults, who have a 30 or higher body weight index (BMI), have been classified as obese in 2010. The weight of the body is divided in pounds by height into inches squared by 703 (weight(lb.)/[height(in)] 2 x 703). By taking these three stages, you may measure your body mass:

- your weight multiplies in pounds by 703.
- your height should be calculated in inches squared.
- The resulting number should be divide from step 1 by the resulting number in step 3.

Obesity may contribute to numerous severe health issues like cardiovascular disease, asthma, stroke, and some cancers.

BENEFITS OF EXERCISE VS. DIET

Combining activity with a balanced lifestyle is more successful than a calorie-restricting approach alone to reduce weight. The symptoms of certain illnesses may be avoided or reversed by exercise. Exercise decreases blood pressure and can be an ideal tool used to avoid a heart attack. Therefore, you are raising the risk to contract other kinds of diseases, such as colon and breast cancer, if you do not exercise. Exercise is often believed to lead to a sense of trust and health, thereby eliminating stress and depression. Exercise is important for weight reduction and weight loss prevention. Exercise will improve your metabolism or the consumption of calories in a day. This will also help you retain and grow lean body fat, which also adds to the additional calories you eat every day.

SIMPLE EXERCISES TO MAXIMIZE FAT LOSS

1. WALKING

Walking is one of the best weight loss exercises — and for a good reason. For beginners, it is convenient and easy to start exercising without feeling overwhelmed or having to buy equipment. It is also a less-impact workout, and the muscles are not strained. According to Harvard Health, a person of 155 pounds (70 kg) is expected to burn about 167 calories at a reasonable speed of 4 miles every 30 minutes. A 12-week study in 20 females with obesity found that averages of 1.5 percent and 1.1 inches (2.8 cm) reduced body fat and waist by walking 50-70 minutes three times per week.

It is easy to implement walking into your everyday routine. Try walking during lunch, taking the stairs instead of the elevator, or taking your dog for extra walks to add more steps to your day. To get started, try to walk 3-4 times a week for 30 minutes. The length or pace of your walks may be slowly improved as you get healthy.

2. JOGGING OR RUNNING

Jogging and running are great exercises for weight loss. Although they seem similar, the main difference is that a jogging pace is usually between 4 – 6 miles per hour (6.4–9.7 miles per hour). Harvard Health estimates that a 155-pound (70-kg) person burns about 298 calories in a 30-minute jogging time at a rate of 5 mph (8-km / h), or 372 calories in a speed of 6 mph (9,7-km / h) for 30-minute running time. In addition, studies have found that jogging and running can contribute to the burning of harmful visceral fat, often called belly fat. This type of fat wraps around your inner organs, and it is associated with different chronic diseases such as heart disease and diabetes.

Jogging and cycling are fantastic workouts that can be done anywhere and are easy to incorporate into your everyday schedule. To get going, try to exercise 3–4 days a week for 20–30 minutes. If you find jogging or outdoor running difficult on your joints, try to run on softer surfaces such as grass. Many treadmills do have adjustable cushioning, which can keep the joints smoother.

3. CYCLING

Cycling is a common workout that will enable you to lose weight and boost your health. While cycling is usually performed outside, several workout centers and gyms have stationary bikes that allow you to cycle whilst remaining inside. Harvard Health estimates that a person that weighs 155 pounds (70-kg) and uses a stationary bike can burn calories at a moderate

rate of about 260 calories per 30 minutes of cycling or 298 calories per 30 minutes on a bike at a moderate rate of 12-13.9 mph (19-22.4 km / h), respectively.

Studies also showed that people with daily workouts have a greater physical health, decreased insulin responsiveness, and a reduced incidence of cardiac failure, stroke, or death than those without frequent cycling. Cycling is perfect for all ranges of people from beginners to competitors. Moreover, it is a non-weight and low-impact workout, and the joints will not be strained much.

How Far Should I Ride a Bike for Weight Loss?

If your bike to lose weight, the duration (the time you expend on biking) is more important than the total distance. That ensures you do not have to fly across the entire Tour de France to pay a couple of pounds. Relieved? You can be, but do not drive the odometer down. Do not turn it off. Go as far as you can.

You may continue your biking training plan with a basic test when you are new to cycling. Using your odometer (or GPS watch or mobile app) to see how fast you are 30 minutes away before you run. Specify the number in the training log and set the goal to the time it takes you to travel down the same path. If the fitness level increases, more miles will be completed in less time, and more calories can be consumed in the process. When you invest more time in the saddle, schedule longer rides throughout the week.

How Fast Should I Cycle to Lose Weight?

If weight loss is your main priority, the pace of exercise is more critical than tempo. A run of higher intensity consumes more calories than a trip of lower intensity. The model of bike you ride and the direction you chose can influence your pace (how intensely you work) and speed (how easily you ride). For starters, you will have to work hard if you ride a heavy mountain bike on muddy off-road trails at 12 miles an hour. But, if you ride on a road bike down a slope, you can almost easily hit the speed.

Learn to use a sensor for heart rate. The system gives a quantitative indicator of how much you work. Try to utilize 70 to 75% of the average heart rate on most drives. When you are not investing in a computer, then use the expected fitness scale. Do you feel like you are operating at level 7 on a scale of 1 to 10 (with 10 being the highest effort)? Can you breathe easily, or are you breathing heavily? Both questions can tell you how hard your body is working.

Where Should I Go Biking to Lose Weight?

The path you chose can have the biggest effect on the number of calories you ingest as it impacts the length and strength. To produce optimal performance, you want to pick a route that helps you to ride reliably at stoplights or intersections without too many breaks. These short breaks cause your heart rate to fall, take too much time to work out, and reduce your riding's calories. Many towns have uninterrupted commuting tracks. Particularly when you start first, choose these safe routes. You do not want to injure yourself by biting off more than you can chew. When you have no connection to a cycle path, it may be worth your time to drive to the spot where there is a long, peaceful lane. You can workout and have some peaceful quiet time to yourself.

The Best Bikes for Weight Loss

The perfect cycle to help you shed weight is the one you use daily. It is important to try every style to find the one that suits your body. Below are some explanations of the different kinds of bikes that you can choose from.

Road Bike

Some cyclists prefer a road bike with thin tires and a smarter environment. A road bike is lightweight, and less energy is needed while riding at a high rate. Road bikes are suitable for asphalt streets and wide, straight stretches of highways. Yet some riders do not feel comfortable on this bike style. A road bike allows you to lean forward slightly when riding. Whether you have back pain or health issues, it might not be your wheel.

Cruiser, Mountain or Cross Bike

You may enjoy the comfort and versatility of a cruiser or mountain bike with heavy, thick tires. Such bikes usually have stability and insulation to make the ride more comfortable. You should usually maintain your body straight while riding this bike type. The thicker pipes also provide greater protection for riders, particularly if they are new to cycling, making them feel safer on these bikes.

Electric Bike

An electric bike (also called an e-bike) might be the right choice for you if you are new to riding or if you want to take your bike on a long day's ride. Brands like Trek render bikes ride like a normal bike, except when you need it, you get a lift. Trek 's Super Commuter promises, for example, a relaxed upright trip with eight separate speeds. When you reach a hill or have a break from difficult pedals, you can use the Bosch pedal assistance feature to maintain speeds of up to 45 km / h.

Recumbent Bike

Some coaches recommend using reclining cycles in the gym, which supports the reclined body to an upright posture, common for normal cycles. Some users, though, prefer a calming cycle for an outdoor trip. Such bikes require you to sit lower to the pavement, typically have a wider saddle, and can fit riders with back difficulties. Because of their low visibility, though, traffic may be harder (and less safe) for these cyclists. Remember where you want to go before you invest in this bicycle style.

4. WEIGHT TRAINING

For people who want to lose weight, weightlifting is a common alternative. According to Harvard Health, an individual of 155 pounds (70 kg) is reported to be burning about 112 calories per 30 minutes of weight exercise.

Weightlifting will also help you develop confidence and promote muscle development that will improve your metabolic rest (RMR) output, or how much calories your body consumes. Another six-month analysis found that only 11 minutes of strength-driven workouts three days a week culminated in an overall metabolic rate rise of 7.4 percent. This rise was equal to the extra 125 calories consumed every day in this analysis. Another research showed that weight training for 24 weeks resulted in a 9 percent improvement in the metabolic rate of males, which led to about 140 more calories burned every day. The metabolic rate raise among women was almost 4%, or 50 more calories a day. However, several experiments have shown that the body goes on losing calories many hours after weight training relative to aerobic exercise.

5. INTERVAL TRAINING

The word interval training, more widely known as HIIT, applies to brief bursts of intense workout, which overlap with rest times. A HIIT exercise usually takes 10-30 minutes and will consume several calories. A research performed in nine healthy people showed that HIIT burnt 25-30 percent more calories per minute than others, such as weightlifting, swimming, and running on a treadmill. This ensures that HIIT will help you eat more calories when you spend less energy.

Numerous studies have also shown that HIIT is especially successful in burning belly fat associated with many chronic diseases. HIIT is simple to incorporate into your workout. You only must choose a form of workouts, such as running, jumping, or riding, and your training and rest times. For starters, pedal as hard as possible for 30 seconds on a bike, followed by a slow pedal for 1 to 2 minutes. Repeat 10–30 minutes of this sequence.

6. SWIMMING

Swimming is a good means of keeping into shape and shedding weight. Harvard Health estimates that a person of 155 pounds (70 kg) burns about 233 calories per half hour. Whether you swim appears to have an effect depends on how many calories you burn. In 30 minutes, a person of 155 pounds brings 298 calories burned in a backstroke, 372 calories burned in a breaststroke, 409 calories burned in a butterfly stroke, and 372 calories burned treading water.

One 12-week study focused on 24 middle-aged women found a significant reduction in body fat, flexibility, and several risk factors, including high total cholesterol and triglycerides in the blood, in body swim 60 minutes 3 times per week. Another bonus to swimming is its low-impact existence, which allows the joints smoother. This makes it a great choice for people suffering from injuries or joint pain.

7. YOGA

Yoga is a common method of exercising and alleviating tension. Although not commonly regarded as a weight-loss exercise, it burns fair quantities of calories and offers many additional health benefits that can lead to weight loss. In fact, the yoga community has enhanced emotional and physical well-being. Besides losing calories, research has shown that yoga will help you to tolerate fatty products, regulate extra food, and better grasp the signs of your body's appetite.

Harvard Health estimates that a person of 155 pounds (70 kg) will burn some 149 calories for 30 minutes of yoga practice. A 12-week study of 60 obese women showed that those who had two 90-minute yoga sessions per week had a greater reduction in the circumference of the waist than the control group, by an average of 1.5 centimeters (3.8 cm). Most fitness facilities provide yoga lessons, but you can do yoga anywhere. This involves the privacy of your own house since several direct tutorials are accessible online.

Yoga Postures for Weight Loss

Yoga can be intended to relax the mind, but it is also a healthy means of forming muscle and shedding weight. Here are several tips that will help you lower the amount on the scale. Keep your posture if you can, which can take you 15-20 seconds at first, but hold up for a few seconds each time you practice and take up to one minute if you can. When required, do one side, and repeat on the other side.

Plank

Keeping straight as a board is one of the best ways to strengthen your core. Maybe it does not appear like it, but it will not take you long to notice it. Subtle modifications will also improve the pressure. Move into a push-up position and hold it for as long as you can. Use that every day to grow hard rock abs.

Warrior II (Virabhadrasana B)

Like a mighty fighter, you should prep your legs and shoulders. Raise your front knee so that your leg is parallel to the ground and get the best out of stance. The longer you can keep it, the closer the quads become.

The secret is calming the mind and breathing. Know, you are a hero! Then, strong fighter, swap sides.

Warrior III (Virabhadrasana C)

Warrior III is the way to go with a more toned core. It is also a perfect way to strengthen your spine, legs, and arms as well as tone your rear end. Contract your abs even more while you hold the position. This does not only allow you to relax; it will even fatten your butt. The longer Warrior III you can hold, the more your booty will benefit.

Triangle (Trikonasana)

Trikonasana does not shake your muscles like other postures but do it regularly, and your abs would be grateful! The torque of trikonasana leads to improved digestion and reduces the accumulation of fat in the abdomen. In fact, you can create more muscle and lose more fat by working the muscles of the legs and arms.

Downward Dog (Adho Mukha Svanasana)

Are you searching for a way to exercise your entire body? Two words: Downward Dog. This moves from a relaxed stance to a revolutionary form of strengthening shoulders, back, and thighs with a little extra focus to other muscles. Take your thigh muscles when you twist them inwards and do the same with your upper arms to get the maximum toning impact. Keep pushing back your palms and feet. Keep it; not stop to breathe! Leave it.

Shoulder Stand (Sarvangasana)

From improved digestion to thyroid therapy and much more energy, the shoulder stand does all that. This inversion improves hormone rates, increasing appetite, enhancing the respiratory mechanism, reinforcing the upper body, legs, and stomach, and allowing you to sleep well. Add this to your routine every day, and you will look like an entirely different human.

Bridge (Setu Bandha Sarvangasana)

Bridge is perfect for the liver, glutes, and weight reduction. The movement you take to your chest massages the thyroid gland softly to generate this essential metabolism-regulating hormone. Tightening down on your foot requires your knees and your back to relax your muscles further. It also serves to relax the gastrointestinal organs and keep the stomach healthy should you need another excuse to play Bridge.

Twisted Chair (Parivrtta Utkatasana)

Call it a Yoga version of a squat — but it is a bit more intense. Parivritta Utkatasana, or the posture of the body, deals for the quads, glutes, and abs. The bending also supports the blood system and the digestive tract. Combine them together with one motion and you have a perfect way to reduce weight.

Bow (Dhanurasana)

Looking for a way to remove bowel fat easily? Bow pose can assist. You will intensify the pose by raising your hands and feet in opposite ways until only your abdomen and pelvis touch the floor. Bow not only allows the abdominal organs to enhance absorption, but it is also an excellent way to strengthen the legs, arms, and back.

Sun Salutations (Surya Namaskara)

You can think of Sun Greetings to make your practice easier. It moves gradually and warms the joints, keeps the blood, and all the positive things going. It does so much more, though. Sun Greetings produce internal heat while also relaxing and toning the essential muscles. You will help cut your hair, ton your muscles, improve your metabolism, and strengthen your digestive system.

8. PILATES

Pilates is a great starting exercise that can help you lose weight. According to a study funded by the American Council, an individual weighing around 140 pounds (64 kg) will eat 108 calories in a Pilates class beginning at 30 minutes, or 168 calories at an advanced class that lasts the same time. While Pilates may not consume as many calories as aerobic exercises, many people find it fun, making it easier for them to stick to it over time. Eight-week research of 37 middle-aged women revealed that the Pilates routine decreased substantially chest, stomach, and hip circumference for 90 minutes 3 days a week, compared with a control group that did not exercise for the same span. Apart from reducing weight, Pilates decreases lower back discomfort and increases strength, coordination, endurance, stamina, and physical health.

If you want to give Pilates a go, try to include it in your weekly routine. You can do Pilates at home or in one of Pilates' many gyms. To further increase weight loss with Pilates, use a healthy diet or other forms of exercise, such as weight training or cardiovascular training.

INCORPORATING EXERCISE INTO YOUR LIFESTYLE

The overall amount of exercise you do during the day is more important than how you do it in a single session or not. That is why small improvements in day-to-day life will make a huge difference.

Healthy lifestyle habits to consider include:

- to move or bike to work or to execute orders.
- Take the stairs rather than the lift.
- Driving further out and walking the remaining distance away from destinations.

NUTRITION AND EXERCISE ARE SIMILARLY VITAL WHEN TRYING TO LOSE WEIGHT

Diet and practice. Those phrases are either disgusting or holy, based on who you refer to. There is no question that they are both vital to good wellbeing, but when it comes to losing weight, do they have equal weight?

The verdict: All the world's exercise won't help you to lose weight if your food is out of hand You know when you're going to spend money here, and a few dollars or doesn't seem like much? Then your credit card declaration and the total sum of your large donor ways are painfully obvious? That is what calories, fat, sodium, and other nutrient information are like, but this is much harder to pinpoint and track than cents and dollars.

Eat Your Way to Happiness, author Elizabeth Somer, MA, R.D., says: "They [dieters] seriously underestimate portions, especially grains and meat... Too many packaged foods, high in calories and poor in oil, salt, sugar and low in carbohydrates, vitamins, minerals, and phytonutrients, are consumed. They eat far too little fresh fruit and vegetables, and when they eat the worst, like potatoes, iceberg lettuce, apple juice, etc." Science reaffirms this claim repeatedly. A recent study by Plos One has been published in

Northern Tanzania, followed by members of a hunter-gatherer tribe. Researchers obtained physical, metabolic, and nutritional data and compared them with the average Western diet of Jack and Jill. They find that the tribe leaders are, in some respect, equal in their eating patterns. They consume just organic, nutritious ingredients, rather than the fat and calorie-laden diets we normally enjoy. The results of the analysis are clear and general. Essentially, you might always run 5 Ks or Sweatin to the Oldies, but it would more definitely be frustrating if you do not adjust the volume and the quantity you consume. To order to remain safe, it is important to follow the trend—not only for a week or a month but for the long term.

NOT SO IMPOSSIBLE

The reasons for the failure of dieters are a million, and the reasons vary from person to person. Men are lying on what they consume, underestimating their calorie consumption by about 700 to 800 calories a day. I think/say that they do even better than they do.

The positive thing is that even such miscalculations are conveniently managed. First, be truthful to yourself. Are you doing the hard work you think you are? If not, please back up. Next, experts recommend dipping actual whole foodstuffs from refined waste. commit at least 75% of your diet to a menu of organic fruit and vegetables, 100% whole grains, legumes, almonds, fatty milk, and seafood. Bring food with you so you will not be tempted by drivers and sellers.

There is no single-size meal schedule. "You ought to plan a lifestyle in which you survive for good, not a fast-fixed trick with the consequence of weight recovery." Respect and love just foodstuffs which will fuel and sustain your body and not products that will harm your wellbeing." So, inquire, do some research, and find a good doctor-supported program that will draw you. Will it be tough? At the beginning, indeed. Normally, every big lifestyle shift is. Was it worth it? Is it worth it? When you get to show off your favorite skinny jeans, you bet it will be worth it.

SIRTFOODS WITH OTHER FOODS

We understand that Sirtfoods and some other foods benefit us, whether its veggies like broccoli or tomatoes, spices like turmeric, or drinks like green tea. The factor these-- and numerous other plant foods-- are great for us, is mostly down to the bio-active plant substances they consist of. For the nutritionally savvy, we may be believing in sulforaphane from broccoli, lycopene from tomatoes, curcumin from turmeric, and catechins from green tea. All the subjects of comprehensive scientific research study that explain simply why these foods are so great for our health.

Rather than simply eating those private foods, as great as they are, what if mixing certain foods-- and therefore their nutrients-- together at meals provided an even larger health boost? What if we could create synergies in various foods between nutrients that maximize their health benefits? This is a new concept, and here are the top 5 examples of how foods can accumulate for optimum results (and you will recognize the sirtfoods in this list).

1. Green tea + lemon

Green tea drinkers can anticipate many health benefits considered that consuming this prized beverage is linked with less cancer, heart diabetes, osteoporosis, and disease. These health advantages can be discussed by its remarkable material of plant compounds called catechins, and especially a type called epigallocatechin gallate (EGCG). Including a capture of lemon juice to your green tea, which is rich in vitamin C, helps to significantly increase the number of catechins that get taken in into the body.

2. Tomato sauce + extra virgin olive oil

The carotenoid of lycopene responsible for the red color of tomatoes is related to a reduction in risk of certain cancers (prostate cancer), cardiovascular disease, osteoporosis and even skin defense against the destructive effects of sunlight. It has been found that cooking and handling tomatoes greatly increases the amount of lycopene the body can consume. Additionally, the existence of fat enhances the synthesis of lycopene. It makes perfect sense to pair your tomato meals with a generous drizzle of extra virgin olive oil.

3. Turmeric+ Black pepper

Turmeric, the ever-present bright yellow spice in standard Indian cooking, is a topic of an extreme clinical study for the anti-cancer characteristics, the potential for lower swelling of the body, and the potential to stave off dementia. Black pepper included increases in its absorption, making it the best double-acting spice. Further aids with curcumin absorption by cooking turmeric in liquid and adding fat.

4. Broccoli + mustard

Broccoli is healthy for us, with advantages like decreased cancer risk, but it is no mystery. Boiling broccoli-especially over boiling-begins to kill the enzyme of myrosinase, which reduces the amount of sulforaphane that can be generated. Adding sulforaphane to other natural sources of myrosinase, such as mustard and horseradish, ensures for those who like their broccoli well-cooked (instead of gently steamed, that 2 to 4 minutes).

5. Salad + Avocado

Lush, leafy vegetables such as kale, spinach, and watercress, are packed with carotenoids that promote health such as immuno-reinforcing lutein and beta-carotene. Once eaten fresh, these carotenoids are more difficult to digest in the form of salads. The addition of some fat can really assist with that, and adding avocado, rich in monounsaturated fat, to a salad, has been revealed to drastically increase the number of carotenoids that can be soaked up.

Take pleasure in the Sirtfoods with additions and gain the included health benefits.

SIRTFOOD SNACKS

Are any beneficial Sirtfood snacks available? Snacking is a term of derogatory connotations that conjures images of confectionary or savory items filled with sugar. To ensure that snacking is an ever-present temptation are never far from our vision, the food market understands our weakest weakness too well, because everything is sweet, and high in fat.

Even if you are prepared to make a healthier choice, it's not obvious why sugar can often be as big for therapies sold as' all-natural' or' no added sugar' as their equivalent for scrap products. The only difference is that the sugars are produced within the naturally sweet components they use instead of being sugarcoated. Look at the label, and you will see that an incredible quantity of sugar can be held off in so-called balanced remedies in the shape of tea, maple syrup, agave, dried fruit (but read on later for more dates), and much more. The upshot is the same— still, a high sugar snack, a lot more costly.

As a result, snacks can typically wind up diminishing the dietary quality of the diet, when they might be a chance to enhance it favorably. So, what should we be snacking on? Are there any sirtfood snacks? There are several of the leading 20 sirtfoods that can be used as the basis for healthy sirtfood snacks.

Nuts must be the stereotypical healthy junk food, packed with 'good' unsaturated fats, plant protein, fiber, and a wealth of vitamins, polyphenols, and minerals. With credentials like that, it is no surprise that is frequently eating nuts slashes the risk of cardiovascular disease. And in comparison, to other heavily fat therapies, nuts are often consumed with a slimmer waistline, probably due to their effective satiating effect. Walnuts, in specific, are an effective sirtuin-activating food and a nice Sirtfood treat. Most importantly, nuts are handbag and workplace desk friendly.

Next in the snacking stakes, and the ideal partner to nuts, is dark chocolate (preferably with an 80-85% cocoa material). Integrate a few squares of dark chocolate with a little handful of nuts, and you have just about the most cardio-protective snack going. Dark chocolate bites are a household favorite considered to be one of the nicest sirtfood snacks as part of the Sirtfood Diet. It integrates a host of polyphenols that promote health into an indulgent treatment. Although the dates of Medjool are obviously very high in sugar (an astounding 66 percent!), ingested moderately, they have no apparent blood glucose rises and is generally correlated with less diabetes and cardiovascular disease because of their exceptional polyphenol content. This makes them one of the healthiest choices for a sweet reward.

Here are nine fast Sirtfood snacks to hit when you need a SIRT boost.

1. Green tea

- 1 cup (200ml)
- 1 of your SIRT 5 a day
- 0 calories

Never underestimate the healthy SIRT increase you can get from a cup of green tea. We suggest at least two cups, have as many cups as you can every day. Not only is green tea SIRT cumulative, but you can also get up to four SIRTs per day when there are four or more cups of green tea.

2. **Red grapes**

- Ten grapes
- One of your SIRT 5 a day
- 30 calories

Another easy way to get one of your SIRT portions and a calorie-friendly snack. Get a punch or two at breakfast or lunch or both in the fridge and grab a couple!

3. **Apples**

- One apple
- One of your SIRT 5 a day
- 47 calories

An apple a day really does keep the doctor away. Reach for an apple as one of your after-lunch easy Sirtfood snacks. It will help keep sugar cravings at bay too.

4. **Cocoa**

- Two tsp/10g cocoa
- One of your SIRT 5 a day
- 33 calories

Try making a chocolate shot with 2 tsp cocoa. 1 tsp sugar and 30ml milk. To make a smooth paste, blend cocoa and sugar with a little hot water from the kettle. Mix the milk together. An instant chocolate hit with just 68 calories (almost).

5. **Olives**

- Six large black or green olives

- One of your SIRT 5 a day
- 75 calories

An afternoon snack or pre-dinner treat for a polyvalent and simple sirtfood. Serve for a full taste at room temperature.

6. Blackberries

- 15 blackberries
- One of your SIRT 5 a day
- 32 calories

Another quick sirtfood to hold in your refrigerator. Superb as a frozen treat.

7. Dark chocolate 85%

- Six squares/20g chocolate
- 1 of your SIRT 5 a day
- 125 calories

Get the hit here with your chocolate! You will need 9 squares/30 g if you want 70% dark chocolate. 180 calories, which will be.

8. Pomegranate seeds

- 50g/half a small pack
- One of your SIRT 5 a day
- 50 calories

Granate seeds bundle up a big SIRT punch simple to be obtained when on the go, and you only need half a 100 g bundle to get one portion of your SIRT.

9. Blueberries

- 25 blueberries (80g)
- One of your sirt five a day
- 36 cals

A few large blueberries could also be one of your quick snacks.

A SIRTFOOD DIET MEAL PLAN

It is described as the kilo-shredding program in news stories which encourages you to drink chocolate and red wine and promises to be like a supermodel and a superhero. On Instagram, it is the stuff UFC featherweight king Conor McGregor does. A few days before his first two big 2016 matches against Nate Diaz, the Irishman took a selfie-and liked over 116,000 users. This is what Adele and Jodie Kidd are doing – so for naysayers, of course, it is just the new fad, another calorie restricting scheme that creates claims that cannot be held.

But the fact is, behind sirt there is much more scientific influence than the usual drop-fat quick scheme. It is based on a class of compounds discovered over the last decade, and recent data shows they are far more significant than commonly believed. So, if the people behind it are correct, we must turn our attention to what we consume.

IS THE SIRT DIET JUST ANOTHER FAD?

What is the evidence? And what is the science behind it all? Science, first. A community of Silent Knowledge Regulator (SIR) proteins – named after Sirt – are proteins that ramp up our metabolism, improve muscle performance, trigger fat burning processes, minimize inflammation and remedy cell damage. Simply placed, sirtuins make us safer, healthier, and milder (there is also proof that they can help battle severe problems like Alzheimer's disease and diabetes, more in the afternoon).

Mild forms of stress – including exercise and calory limitation – trigger the body's sirtuin production, but recent discoveries have found that chemicals known in fruit and vegetables as sirtuin activators can do the same. Sirt foods as called by diet makers Aidan Goggins and Glen Matten – are especially high in those sirtuin activators. The theory is that you will lose fat and improve your health when eating a diet made up of those foods. Goggins and Matten created the Sirt Plan, the 7-day meal program, to check the theory. This is made easy: the regular intake of calories for the first three days is reduced to 1.000 and consists of three grassy juices and a meal rich in Sirtfood. The consumption of calories is raised to 1.500 on days four to seven and is composed of two drinks and two meals. After the first week, a healthy diet full of Sirt foods and more green juices would be prescribed. This sounds terrible on the face of it: even most quick diets give more calories.

Rannoch Donald, a coach and teacher who pursued the diet, says: "I felt at all challenging. The juice is essential: it is like the fuel of a rocket. The first week was accompanied by easy sailing, during which I was 5 kg lighter for three weeks. But more notably, in a few years, I thought the strongest I have had. I was reducing my body weight; I was happier eating; I did not have any issues with the body; I felt healthy. I was studying, practicing, and fantastically healing a half dozen lessons a week from even the most horrible session in Brazil."

Goggins and Matten hired 37 people from XK Gym, including 15 overweight, to check the diet in a broader context. All these workouts were mild, none were through, and only some continued to do fewer. And the tests were surprising after just one week, even with the calorie limitation: the participants lost a total of 3 kg of weight but instead placed on only 0.8 kg of muscle. You should hope to lose an average of 1 kg from a normal diet that lowers the calories in a week to the same amount.

WHY IS SIRT NOT AVAILABLE?

There is the obvious question: if sirtuins improve too much, why are pharmaceutical firms not rushing to pill it into a type of supplement? Short reply: since they still do not grasp the process by which they function entirely, their materials would not always be as easily consumed by the body as the normal types. Goggins and Matten point to the resveratrol example: "In fact, its absorption by the body is low, but its bioavailability (How much the body can use) is at least six times higher than its natural food matrix of red wine. We agree that it's healthier to consume a large variety of such nutrients in the form of natural whole foods that coexist with the hundreds of other bioactive chemical plants, which function in a synergistic manner to improve our wellbeing."

FAST AND FURIOUS?

This is, of course, the part of the sirt diet which criticizes. Usually, the program relies in the early stages on calorie restriction, at least, so the weight reduction of more than 1 kg a week is, according to prior practice, unsafe or unrealistic. This is a legitimate concern: early lack of calories appears to come from calorie depletion and reduced water fluctuation in the majority of diets for calories and, as recently studied by participants in The Biggest Loser reveals, rationing yourself will slow your metabolism down every day to an almost permanent crawl.

But that's not what sirt does, Goggins and Matten answer. Yeah, the diet represents certain facets of fasting, and sirt foods tend to turbo-charge the impact of a calorie limit for the first seven days of the maximum diet. But it is a little tougher than being looking for short-term improvements. And how does that work? Why does it work? Ok, firstly, the "energy" part of the equation must be grasped. "Everyone in their lives needs a certain amount of stress," says Goggins. "We build tension on the body every time we exercise, which can be a positive or a bad thing. There are temptations to work hard still, to strive harder.

However, this carries the risk of excessively stressed growth; this carries the risk of burnout and weakening immune systems. "The other side: you can improve the capacity of the body to deal with higher rates of stress while subjected to higher levels of stress. "Animal stress reactions are probably more developed than our own," Goggins says. "Think about it: we can go to the hungry and thirsty for food and drink; we consider shade too hot; we can run from assaults. The plants, on the other side, are stagnant and must tolerate many of these physiological pressures and risks. Over the past billions of years, they have therefore built a highly sophisticated stress response mechanism that humiliates [human beings], creating an enormous array of natural vegetable chemical products – called polyphenols – that allows them to adjust and thrive effectively to their climate. When we eat these plants, we eat the nutrients of polyphenols, which cause our own inherent mechanisms of stress reaction. We are talking almost the same path as fasting and exercising – sirtuins.

According to Goggins, polyphenols are the one item that the traditional American diet has plenty, so when excluded from the diet, the much-valued Mediterranean diet lacks almost complete efficacy. Via mermaids, polyphenols may be used to imitate Brown Adipose tissue ("good" fat that helps to produce body heat) across a variety of weight loss results, including promoting white adipose tissue (traditionally poor stuff). They also assist with fullness problems by increasing the response of the body to the satiety hormone leptin.

"These natural plant compounds are often labeled 'calorie-restrictive mimetic' as they can alter the beneficial results of the fasting in our cells, such as fat burning," says Goggins. "The results are shifting the game. Although we have more sophisticated signaling molecules than our own, the effects are comparable to what we would do alone.

THE REAL HEALTH FOODS

Sirt often has more than the makeup of the bone. In addition to the experiments by Goggins and Matten, more scientifically monitored studies on Sirtfoods yielded positive performance. In October 2015, for example, Columbia University researchers in New York noticed the dissolution of drinking water in 19 intermediate-age topics with a gram of cacao, particularly rich in sirtuin-enhanced epicatechin. In November of the same year, Monash University researchers in Melbourne recorded that, if patients in the early phases of type 2 diabetes applied a gram of turmeric a day to their diets, their working memory increased. There are some indications for people with diabetes that sirtuin activation raises the volume of insulin that can be secreted and makes it function more efficiently. In the skeleton, sirtuins promote osteoblast growth and preservation, a cell group responsible for the formation of new bones.

When more work is carried out, the next big thing for Sirt will be the connection to leucine, the leading muscle builder in the branched-chain amino acids (BCAAs). Leucine is a main protein synthesis regulator and stimulates a protein called mTOR (although you do not have to think about it to grasp the next bit). "Leucine is a blade with two sides," Goggins says. "It's muscle accelerator, but if you don't have the internal machines to handle, the engine will explode." Theoretically, having a heavier sirt food diet can increase your body's protein content so that it can successfully absorb the old recommendation "20-30 g a sitting" into the past.

All this, of course, needs further work. Thirty-seven participants in one research gym and other experiments on the effect of sirtuins on animals or human cells have been performed – and neither expected to reflect what occurs inside the body accurately. But despite all skepticism of the more extreme arguments of food, by adopting a variant of the Sirt Plan, it is difficult to see what you are to sacrifice. Although you would not put up the calorie-limited version of the diet and go right into the "maintenance" phase, in the so-called Blue Zones, places of the world such as Sardinia and

Okinawa, where people live longer and healthier lives, you would have eaten a wide variety of foods. "I don't like the word diet, so this is a lifestyle plan rather than a quick-fire operation," Donald says. "It's just healthy health. Yet, with the introduction of green juice cocktails, the general approach remains to integrate balanced whole-of-life products rather than to deify 'superfoods.'" Or, to put it another way: you will not get happier unless more spinach, tomatoes, walnuts, yet red wine are introduced. Particularly though you are not a UFC or a supermodel fighter.

THE MEAL PLAN

With these values, here is what should be on the menu during the maintenance process over a week (green juices aside).

BREAKFAST:

- Fruit smoothie made with rolled oats and soy milk
- Kale omelet
- Muesli, yogurt and blueberries

LUNCH AND DINNER:

- Rocket salad with tuna, tomatoes and cucumber dressed in olive oil
- Grilled fish with buckwheat salad
- Veggie-packed spicy tofu stir fry with birds-eye chili
- Chicken and soba noodle stir fry
- Kale salad with edamame beans and red onion dressed in olive oil
- Tofu burgers with wholegrain bread and salad
- Spicy chicken curry served with wholegrain brown rice

SNACKS:

- Walnuts
- Coffee
- Celery and hummus
- Dark chocolate
- Fresh fruit, particularly strawberries, apples and oranges

LEAN GENE

Genetics is a long-standing beat-up excuse. Therefore, people are lazy, weak, and behave as though they do not realize what is going on in their lives. Yeah, certain mutations may render you predisposed to a disease, but that does not indicate that you get older. It also ensures that you can grow a good gene in life and not build poor habits. It means that you can build as strong an atmosphere as you can to prevent inherited vulnerabilities.

It appears like biology is the direction our scientific world shifts. This is terrifying to me. Essentially, our chromosomes are what create you and me. If the right genetic code somewhere, we could all be the same. The obesity gene was long known, but just recently did it reveal how this gene functions. I named the FTO mutation, and mice who had not pigged the mutation were slouched all day long and miraculously appeared healthier. It seems like the right cure for individuals to do or feed properly. Any other study has shown that individuals with this amazing FTO gene have an excess of 7 pounds heavier and 70% heavier likely to be obese. 70% is a big amount. Either we have individuals who will not want to remain alive, or this gene is just an end to all genes. My guess is that people do not want to remain safe.

Mice are really like us when it comes to our genes and DNA, and the experiments performed on this mouse will demonstrate how we accumulate any extra weight from this FTO mutation. To pharmaceutical firms, this is a major move. Their number is projected to be 400 million obese in the world and is rising. 2 of them are overweight here in states for every three men. These figures are bad, but they get worse. This indicates that something about the program is incorrect. All need to be changed.

Being obese raises any risk factor that you could think about. If you must bear this additional weight, your body faces a lot more pain than normal. Imagine wearing a dumbbell weighing around 50 pounds anywhere you go.

Such studies will ultimately contribute to obesity care. They view obesity as a disorder and not as a preference for lifestyle. People may lose weight; the FTO gene may or may not lose weight. Some will consider it difficult, but it is always feasible. I can see the future. I will see the future. When the first advert on television speaks about the consequences of the FTO mutation, they inquire if you are fat with certain alarming figures, then then the main selling advertisement on whatever the medication is.

My biggest pet peeve is this. Why are we investigating this? Yeah, for the sake of information, it is necessary and can be achieved, but why not look to the past where the citizens are not fat? See if they were slim, what they were drinking and how they were sleeping. We will avoid researching illness in pursuit of wellness—health research to determine fitness. Look at mature cultures that do not involve illness or disease. Look at how strong and slim they were.

Thus, my aim is to avoid researching illness to pursue wellness. Do not allow your chromosomes to dictate who you are and how you are. Your climate and biology play an important role, and I think it plays a more important role. You can improve yourself, whether it be autism, a professional athlete, success in school or some other reason. You should do it, whether it is healthy genes or not.

DO YOU HAVE LEAN GENES?

What is your genetic weight? Just 5% of all weight disorders compensate for obesity genes. About 95% of the weight issues are due to chromosomes. This fact has not affected our culture's high incidence of obesity. Nor should we blame the issue of obesity on high-fat diets. Because fat contains nine calories per gram, unlike the carbs or protein that only contains four calories per gram, our crisis still cannot be nailed to fat consumption. Evidence has demonstrated, in addition, that low-fat diets do not work well and do more damage than good. And to add to that – it is not a major determinant of body fat to avoid fat in your diet. The Women's Wellness Project, the first diet and body weight research study, showed that 50,000 people have no substantial loss in weight in low-fat diets.

Were you conscious that you may potentially be at an "ideal" weight that looks fine and severely obese? We refer to it as "Skinny Fat." Many models who you find to be slim or lean will potentially have a large proportion of body fat. Anything higher than 30% is clinically obese. Some of these "ideal" images have very little lean mass on their frames. As we always claim, they are simply just skin and bones, and we must often have fat under the skin in our definition. This is important to learn what the real body fat or muscle fat percentage is. This marker determines not only your real slimness but also your actual health. That is why I still suggest that you check your fat body composition.

Without the specific check – the main avoidance of slipping into the 'skinny fat' group is a full and healthy diet. Here is a trick-because you have a higher rating, you will consume better. If you have more lean muscle mass than you must burn fewer to sustain your weight, you will potentially consume more calories. Your body is a robotic oven that can break down everything you consume quickly – comfortably. Not that it burns all down quickly. If you feed unhealthy foods on your body, your muscle mass reduces, and the capacity to lose calories is therefore popular. There are two main things that improve lean muscle mass-exercise resistance and protein. Both inappropriate proportions for your body type and your workout intensity should give you the perfect fat, lean muscle ratio.

Turning to the topic of obesity and weight care, the main aspect is to personalize the strategy. We learn more and more about something named Nutrigenomics in my area of agriculture. It is the awareness of how we can affect our genes through food. Yeah, this right has been learned-our diet will affect and probably alter the expression of our genome. Whether you like, let us name it Genetic Eating. When we supply the body with building blocks and good nutrients, the genes "turn on" as it were. Put simply-you come into this world with some genetic makeup, and if you do not properly "feed" your genes-the the healthy expression of our genes is stopped. Of examples, let us refer to it as the "good weight gene" without the proper nutrients that this gene shuts down. To switch the genetic light on, we will send our body the correct current (a little wordplay)-and it works. This is, of reality, a very basic description for a very complicated operation. The most important aspect you can realize is that you should adjust your DNA to blend in with your clothes, so YOUR Food is one of the most important functions.

HEALTH BENEFITS OF SIRTFOODS

There is proof that sirtuin activators may provide a wide variety of health benefits as well as muscle strengthening and appetite suppression. That involves better memory, better control of blood sugar levels in the body, and the clearance of damage caused by free radical molecules that build up in cells and result in cancer and other diseases.

'The positive effects of the intake of food and beverages rich in sirtuin activators in decreasing chronic disease risk are important observational evidence,' said Professor Frank Hu, an authority on diet and epidemiology at Harvard University in a recent paper in Advances In Nutrition. An anti-aging diet is particularly suited to a Sirt food diet. While the entire plant realm is home to sirtuin activators, only some fruits and vegetables have enough to report to Sirtfood. Examples include green tea, cacao powder, Indian spice pea, spinach, onion, and parsley.

In many stores, fruit, and vegetables such as strawberries, avocados, bananas, spinach, kiwis, broccoli, and pep are quite low inactivators for sirtuins. This does not mean, however, that they are not worth eating because they have many other advantages.

The advantage of a Sirtfood-packed diet is that it is much more versatile than other diets. You could just consume a few Sirt foods healthily. Or you could concentrate on them. The 5:2 menu could require more calories on low-calorie days by incorporating Sirt foods. One notable observation of a Sirtfood diet trial is that participants lose excessive weight without weakening their muscles. It was also reasonable for participants to build weight, contributing to a more formed and toned body. It is the beauty of Sirtfoods: fat burning is activated, but muscle growth, maintenance and repair are promoted. In comparison to other foods, weight reduction typically occurs from fat and muscle, which speeds down the digestion of the body and allows weight to rebound more easily.

ARE THERE ANY OTHER BENEFITS TO SIRTFOODS?

Sirtuins have a hand in several other safety advantages as well. Included:

Sleep

Activating sirtuins adds to improve the circadian cycle such that you generate hormones while you are expected to improve sleep and rise.

Diabetes

Sirtuins allow cells more responsive to insulin so that they can lose more blood glucose. As the key to both diabetes and weight gain is insulin resistance, there can be just positive news for the waistline.

Memory

Turmeric boosts short-term performance and defends against cognitive disorders. Pack your morning juice to begin the day with a brainier.

55 SIRTFOOD DELICIOUS RECIPES

1. SIRTFOOD BITES

INGREDIENTS:

- (85% cocoa solids), 1 ounce (30g) dark chocolate, 1/4 cup cocoa nibs or broken into pieces;
- 1 cup (120g) walnuts
- pitted, 9 ounces (250g) Medjool dates
- One tablespoon ground turmeric
- One tablespoon cocoa powder
- the scraped seeds of 1 vanilla pod or one teaspoon vanilla extract
- One tablespoon extra virgin olive oil
- 1 to 2 tablespoons of water

INSTRUCTIONS:

1. Place the walnuts and the chocolate in a food processor and then Proceed until you've got a fine powder.
2. Add all other ingredients other than water and combine until a ball is shaped. Depending on the consistency of the mixture, you may or may not add the water — you don't want that to be too adhesive.
3. Formake a bite-sized paste with your hands and cool down for at least 1 hour in an airtight jar before consuming them.
4. You can roll some of the balls to a different finish if you want to in some cocoa or dried cocoa. And can be store in your fridge for up to one week.

2. SIRT SUPER SALAD

INGREDIENTS:

- 1 3⁄4 ounces (50g) endive leaves
- 1 3⁄4 ounces (50g) arugula
- 3 1⁄2 ounces (100g) smoked salmon slices
- 1⁄2 cup (50g) celery including leaves, sliced
- 1⁄2 cup (80g) avocado, peeled, stoned, and sliced
- 1⁄8 cups (15g) walnuts, chopped
- 1⁄8 cup (20g) red onion, sliced
- One tablespoon capers
- One tablespoon extra virgin olive oil
- One large Medjool date, pitted and chopped
- juice of 1⁄4 lemon
- 1⁄4 cup (10g) parsley, chopped

INSTRUCTIONS:

1. In a plate or wide cup, position the salad leaves.
2. Mix all the remainder of the ingredients and pour over the seeds.

3. MISO-MARINATED BAKED COD WITH STIR-FRIED GREENS AND SESAME

INGREDIENTS:

- One tablespoon extra virgin olive oil
- 3 1⁄2 teaspoons (20g) miso
- One tablespoon mirin
- 1⁄8 cup (20g) red onion, sliced
- 1 x 7-ounce (200g) skinless cod fillet
- Two garlic cloves, finely chopped
- 3⁄8 cup (40g) celery, sliced
- One teaspoon finely chopped fresh ginger
- One Thai chili, finely chopped
- 3⁄4 cup (50g) kale, roughly chopped
- 3⁄8 cup (60g) green beans
- Two tablespoons (5g) parsley, roughly chopped
- One teaspoon sesame seeds
- 1⁄4 cup (40g) buckwheat
- One tablespoon tamari (or soy sauce, if not avoiding gluten)
- One teaspoon ground turmeric

INSTRUCTIONS:

1. Combine the miso, mirin and one oil tea cubicle. Rub the whole cod and set for 30 minutes to marinate. Oven heated to 220 degrees C (425 degrees F).
2. Bake the cod for 10 minutes.
3. Heat the remaining oil in a large frying pan or wok. Remove the celery, garlic, chili, ginger, green beans, and kale and deep fry for a few minutes. Sprinkle and sprinkle until the kale is soft and baked. To help the cooking process, you might have to put a bit of water into the pot.
4. Cook buckwheat together with turmeric in accordance with the package instructions.
5. Serve the stir-fry with sesame, parsley and tamari seeds and fish. Serve in the stir-fry.

4. AROMATIC CHICKEN BREAST WITH KALE, RED ONIONS, TOMATO, AND CHILI SALSA

INGREDIENTS:

- Skinless 1⁄4 pound (120 g), Monotonous chicken breast.
- Two ground turmeric teaspoons
- 1/2 lemon juice
- Extra virgin olive oil one charcoal tablespoon.
- Three-quarters (50 g) kale, cut off.
- Red onion cut 1⁄8 cup (20 g)
- New ginger sliced with one teaspoon
- 1⁄3 cup of light wheat (50 g);

The Salsa

- One small (130 g) tomato
- One Thai chili, deeply sliced.
- One caper of a teaspoon, fine cut
- Parsley 2 teaspoons (5 g), fine cut
- 1⁄4 lemon of juice

INSTRUCTIONS:

1. Remove the eye from the tomato to make the salsa and pinch it finely, ensuring that the fluid remains as high as possible. Combine chile, capers, lemon juice and parsley. You might mix it all in, but the end product is a little different.
2. Oven to 220 degrees Celsius (425 ° F), in one teaspoon, marinate the chicken breast with a little oil and lemon juice. Leave for five to ten minutes.
3. Then add the marinated chicken and cook on either side for about a minute, until pale golden, transfer to the oven (on a baking tray, if your pan is not ovenproof), 8 to 10 minutes or until cooked. Remove from the oven, cover with tape, and wait until eaten for five minutes.
4. Cook the kale for 5 minutes in a steamer in the meantime, in a little butter, fry the red onions and the ginger and then mix in the

fluffy but not browned chalk.
5. Cook the buckwheat with the remaining turmeric teaspoon according to the package instructions. Eat rice, tomatoes and salsa. Eat together.

5. ASIAN SHRIMP STIR-FRY WITH BUCKWHEAT NOODLES

INGREDIENTS:

- Two teaspoons tamari (you can use soy sauce if you are not avoiding gluten)
- 1⁄3 pound (150g) shelled raw jumbo shrimp, deveined
- Two teaspoons extra virgin olive oil
- Two garlic cloves, finely chopped
- Three ounces (75g) soba (buckwheat noodles)
- One teaspoon finely chopped fresh ginger
- One Thai chili, finely chopped
- 1⁄2 cup (45g) celery including leaves, trimmed and sliced, with leaves set aside
- 1⁄8 cup (20g) red onions, sliced
- 3⁄4 cup (50g) kale, roughly chopped
- 1⁄2 cup (75g) green beans, chopped
- 1⁄2 cup (100ml) chicken stock

INSTRUCTIONS:

1. Prepare the pan for high heat, then cook the shrimps for 2 to 3 minutes in 1 tamari tea cubicle and one olive tea cubicle.
2. Switch to a tray of shrimp. Cover the pan with a towel or cloth, and you'll need it again.
3. Cook the noodles 5 to 8 minutes or as indicated on the box in boiling water. Drain and reserve. Drain.
4. Fried in the remaining tamari and oil over half to high heat for 2 to 3 minutes in the garlic, pepper, ginger and red onion, celery (but not the blade). Stir the stock and boil until they are tender, but always crunchy, then simmer for a minute or two.
5. Stir in a pan and put back to boil, then take the shrimp, pasta, and celery leaves from the oven, and drink.

6. ASIAN SHRIMP STIR-FRY WITH BUCKWHEAT NOODLES

INGREDIENTS:

- Two teaspoons tamari (you can use soy sauce if you are not avoiding gluten)
- 1/3 pound (150g) shelled raw jumbo shrimp, deveined
- Two teaspoons extra virgin olive oil
- Two garlic cloves, finely chopped
- 3 ounces (75g) soba (buckwheat noodles)
- One teaspoon finely chopped fresh ginger
- 1 Thai chili, finely chopped
- 1/2 cup (45g) celery including leaves, trimmed and sliced, with leaves set aside
- 1/8 cup (20g) red onions, sliced
- 3/4 cup (50g) kale, roughly chopped
- 1/2 cup (75g) green beans, chopped
- 1/2 cup (100ml) chicken stock

INSTRUCTIONS:

1. Cover the pot over high heat and cook the shrimp for 2-3 minutes in 1 tamari tablespoon and one teaspoon of butter.
2. Move to a plate the shrimp. Remove the saucepan with a cloth, as you will use the towel again.
3. Cook the noodles 5 to 8 minutes or as indicated on the box in boiling water, drain and hold.
4. In the meantime, sauce on medium to high heat for 2 to 3 minutes, fry the garlic, chili, ginger, red onion, celery (not the leaves), green beans and chalk in the remaining tamari, oil. Add the stock and carry it to the boil and simmer until the vegetables are crunchy and cooked for a minute or two.
5. Add the pan with shrimp, noodles and celery leaves, bring back to the boil and serve off the heat.

7. STRAWBERRY BUCKWHEAT TABBOULEH

INGREDIENTS:

- One tablespoon ground turmeric
- 1⁄3 cup (50g) buckwheat
- 1⁄2 cup (80g) avocado
- 1⁄8 cup (20g) red onion
- 3⁄8 cup (65g) tomato
- One tablespoon capers
- 1⁄8 cup (25g) Medjool dates, pitted
- 2⁄3 cup (100g) strawberries, hulled
- 3⁄4 cup (30g) parsley
- juice of 1⁄2 lemon
- One tablespoon extra virgin olive oil
- 1 ounce (30g) arugula

INSTRUCTIONS:

1. Cook the turmeric with buckwheat according to the directions for the box.
2. Rinse to cool off.
3. Chop the agua finely, peppers, red onions, bananas, capers, and pots, and blend along with the fresh buckwheat.
4. Dice the strawberries and combine the oils with the lemon juice softly in the salad. Serve on arugula bed.

8. SIRTFOOD GREEN JUICE

INGREDIENTS:

- a large handful (1 ounce or 30g) arugula
- Two large handfuls (about 2 1/2 ounces or 75g) kale
- 2 to 3 large celery stalks (5 1/2 ounces or 150g), including leaves
- a very small handful (about 1/4 ounce or 5g) flat-leaf parsley
- 1/2- to 1-inch (1 to 2.5 cm) piece of fresh ginger
- 1/2 medium green apple
- 1/2 level teaspoon matcha powder
- juice of 1/2 lemon

INSTRUCTIONS:

1. Mix the greens together and then sauté the greens. We discovered that the efficiency of juicers could vary greatly from leafy food to rejuicate the rest of the food, and before moving to other ingredients. The goal is to get approximately 2 or 1/4 cup of green juice or around two fluid ounces.
2. Celery juice, apple, ginger juice
3. You can peel and place the citrus fruit also, but it is much easier just to squeeze the citrus fruits by hand into the juice. By this point, you should have a limit of about 1 cup (250 ml) of water.
4. You just add the matcha if the juice is cooked and ready to drink. Into a glass, add a small amount of the juice and mix with a blaze or teaspoon vigorously.
5. Add the rest of the juice when the matcha is dissolved. Give it a quick swirl, and then drink your tea. Feel free to enhance the palate of plain water.

9. SIRT MUESLI (SERVES 1)

To make it in bulk or to make it overnight, simply put the dry ingredients together and store it in a container. Only apply the strawberries and yogurt the next day, and it is ready to go.

INGREDIENTS:

- 10g buckwheat puffs
- 20g buckwheat flakes
- 100g strawberries, hulled and chopped
- 15g coconut flakes or desiccated coconut
- 15g walnuts, chopped
- 40g Medjool dates, pitted and chopped
- 10g cocoa nibs
- 100g plain Greek yogurt (or vegan alternative, such as soya or coconut yogurt)

INSTRUCTIONS:

1. Put together all these products (leave the fruits and yogurt out if you do not instantly serve).

10. MATCHA WITH VANILLA

Swap the tasty green matcha and the white tea in this Japanese-style tea or coffee. It is easy to make at home, and it only takes 5 minutes

INGREDIENTS:

- seeds from half a vanilla pod
- ½ tsp matcha powder

INSTRUCTION:

1. Heat the kettle then apply 100ml of water to it. In a tiny cup, pour half the hot tea, steam and then transfer the matcha powder and vanilla seeds to the remainder of the bottle.
2. Stir the mixture up to a smooth, slightly smooth and lump-free matcha with a bamboo whisk or mini-electric whisk. In a hot teapot, throw the water away and then dump the cooked matcha tea into it.

11. TURMERIC TEA

Take the spice rack and catch turmeric to create this coffee-free drink. This orange spice occurs everywhere on the menus

INGREDIENTS:

- 1 tbsp fresh grated ginger
- 3 heaped tsp ground turmeric
- honey or agave and lemon slices, to serve
- One small orange, zest pared

INSTRUCTIONS:

1. Boil in a pot 500ml of tea. Into a teapot or jug, put turmeric, ginger and orange-pink. Sprinkle with the heating water for about 5 minutes.
2. Strain into two cups using a sieve or Tea strainer, apply a slice of lemon and sweeten, whether you prefer, with sweet honey or agave.

12. DATE AND WALNUT CINNAMON BITES

These cinnamon dates and walnut bites are quick to whip for a good snack. They act even as a reward when you have friends

INGREDIENTS:

- Three pitted Medjool dates
- Three walnut halves
- Add the ground cinnamon, to taste

INSTRUCTION:

1. Split each walnut half carefully into three pieces and then do the same with the dates. Place on top of every date a piece of walnut and cover with cinnamon dust.

13. RED CHICORY, PEAR AND HAZELNUT SALAD

INGREDIENTS:

For the dressing

- 1 tsp sherry or cider vinegar
- Two heads of red chicory or white if not available
- 25g hazelnuts, toasted and chopped
- Two ripe red Williams pears a good handful of rocket leaves
- 2 tbsp hazelnut or olive oil
- 1 tsp green peppercorns in brine, optional
- 2 tbsp. of salad oil, either sunflower oil or oil with safflower.

INSTRUCTIONS:

1. Dress up. If they use green pepper beans, lightly crush them in a bowl or use a pestle and mortar with a wooden spoon. Mix the oils and vinegar and sprinkle with the salt.
2. Remove the stalk from the chicory and remove any cute or tired external leaves. Break the leaves carefully and organize 5-6 in 4 sections-whether each one is big, cut or tear.
3. Take the tongs out of the pears, and lengthwise quarter the pears. Cut the kernel and dice the fruit thinly. Arrange the chicory slices and spoon more than half of the sauce. Pour over the rocket the remaining dressing and salt and pepper season. Place the leaves on top of each salad and easily flip. Sprinkle and top with almonds.

14. ITALIAN KALE

This vibrant green lateral dish was tasted and dressing in vinegar, giving it a sweet and sour taste, which keeps you coming back for longer.

INGREDIENTS:

- Three tbsp red wine vinegar
- Three garlic cloves, finely sliced
- Three tbsp olive oil
- 300g cavolo nero or kale, roughly shredded

INSTRUCTIONS:

1. Then apply the vinegar and a splash of water to heat the oil into a large bowl with a plate, fill it with garlic.
2. Top up the kale and cover the steam, adding more water if the pot gets too dry for 4-5 minutes. Season with a little salt of the sea once wilted.

15. BROCCOLI AND KALE GREEN SOUP

This super healthy soup combines broccoli with ginger, coriander, and turmeric to make a dense and fat lunch with nutrients.

INGREDIENTS:

- One tbsp sunflower oil
- 500ml, by mixing powder of 1 tbsp broth and boiling water in a jug
- Two garlic cloves, sliced
- Sliced ½ tsp ground coriander, thumb-sized piece ginger.
- Piece 3 cm / 1 in the fresh, fresh root of turmeric, peeled and grated or 1⁄2 tsp.
- 85g broccoli100g kale, chopped
- 200g courgettes, roughly sliced
- One lime, zested and juiced
- A thin, finely chopped parsley pack with a few whole leaves.

INSTRUCTIONS

1. In a deep pot place the butter, add the garlic, ginger, coriander, salt and turmeric, fry over medium heat for 2 minutes, then add 3 tbsp of water, give the spices a little more moisture.
2. Add the courgettes, ensure that the slices have a good mixture of all the spices, then cook 3 minutes. Add stock of 400 ml and cook for 3 minutes.
3. Add the remaining stock to the broccoli, kale and lime juice. Let all vegetables soft and cook once more for 3-4 minutes.
4. Remove the heat and add the pickled parsley. Load it all into a machine and blend it easily to high speed. It'll be a pretty leaf with patches of shadow (the kale). Decorate with parsley and lime.

16. STRAWBERRY, TOMATO AND WATERCRESS SALAD WITH HONEY & PINK PEPPER DRESSING

As a side meal, or even for lunch on your own, eat this cherry, tomato, and aquarelle salad. Pink peppers offer a gentle spice in the dressing

INGREDIENTS:

- 100g watercress, woody stalks discarded
- 300g strawberries
- Three tbsp extra virgin olive oil
- Two strawberries (about 40g), chopped
- For the dressing
- Three tbsp pink peppercorns
- ½ lemon, juiced
- ½ tbsp honey
- 250g mixed tomatoes

INSTRUCTIONS:

1. Toast the potatoes with a dry pot for 1-2 minutes, then cook quickly with a stick and a touch of Salt to split up the skins.
2. To prepare the sauce. Attach and crush the two strawberries into a paste.
3. Stir in the lemon juice and the honey. In a large bowl, put the dressing and the olive oil whisk. Please check the seasoning and if you like, add a bit more salt or lemon juice. To assemble the bowl, split the strawberries into quarters or thin wedges, and finely slice the tomatoes, chopping some and halving others, so you get plenty of various shapes. In the bowl, mix with the hammer.
4. Place the salad on a tray, or layer the salad between four pots. Spoon over the left clothes in the tub.

17. ORIENTAL SALMON AND BROCCOLI TRAY BAKE

Everything you need to create this Asian flavored fish dish with balanced greens and fresh lemon is five ingredients

INGREDIENTS:

- One head broccoli, broken into florets
- Four skin-on salmon fillets
- juice ½ lemon, ½ lemon quartered
- Two tbsp soy sauce
- small bunch spring onions, sliced

INSTRUCTIONS:

1. 180C/160C heating stove/gas 4. Place the salmon in a large tin of roasts, making space for each fillet.
2. Wash and dry broccoli and arrange around the fillets, while still a little wet. Place overall the lemon water, then apply the quarter of a lemon.
3. Sprinkle half the onions with a little olive oil and add them to the oven for 14 minutes. Sprinkle it with the soy, detach from the oven, return for another 4 minutes to the oven before salmon is fried. Just before serving, sprinkle with the remaining spring onions.

18. SUPERHEALTHY SALMON SALAD

Super-healthy by word, super-healthy by nature: This salad is rich in omega-3, iron and calcium and counts as 2 of your five a day salad.

INGREDIENTS:

- Two salmon fillets
- 100g couscous
- 1 tbsp olive oil
- juice one lemon
- 200g sprouting broccoli, roughly shredded, larger stalks removed
- a small handful of pumpkin seeds
- seeds from half a pomegranate
- Two handfuls watercress
- olive oil and extra lemon wedges, to serve

INSTRUCTION:

1. Heat a stage steamer with gas. Season the couscous, then sprinkle with 1 tsp oil. Pour water over the couscous and cover it by 1 cm, then set aside. When the water in the steamer hits the simmer, tip the broccoli into the water and then place the salmon in the above stage—Cook for 3 minutes before the salmon is finished, and tender broccoli. Drain the broccoli and refrigerate under the cool spray.
2. Add the remaining oil and lemon juice together. Toss the broccoli, pomegranate seeds and the pumpkin seeds with the lemon dressing through the couscous. Chop the watercress loosely at the last minute, then throw into the couscous. Serve, if you want, with the tuna, lemon wedges to squeeze over and fresh olive oil to drizzle.

19. MALABAR PRAWNS

Create one of the favorite dishes of Kerala-Malabar prawns, a South Indian coast specialty. They are fast and easy to prepare and filled with distinct flavors

INGREDIENTS:

- 400 grams of frozen king prawns2 tsp turmeric
- Kashmiri chili powder 3-4 tsp.
- Lemon juice of 4 tsp, with a pinch
- 40gm ginger, half peeled and dried, half finely cut in similar lines
- Vegetable oil 1 tbsp
- Four Leaves of curry
- Two - Four orange, half and desirable chilies
- One fine-sliced onion
- One tsp black pepper cracked
- 40gm new rubbed coconut
- 1/2 batch of coriander, leaves only

INSTRUCTIONS:

1. Wash the prawns in cold water, then dry pick. Toss them and put aside with the turmeric, chili powder, lemon juice, and grated ginger.
2. Heat the oil in a saucepan and add the curry leaves, chili, ginger sliced and onion. Cook for around 10 mins until translucent, then apply the black pepper.
3. Stir-fry the prawns with some marinade once tender, around 2 minutes. Season and apply a squeeze of lemon juice if necessary. Serve with coconut and leaves of coriander added.

20. CHICKEN, KALE AND SPROUT STIR-FRY

Brussels sprouts are not enough for Christmas-add them for extra protein and crunch in a balanced noodle dish

INGREDIENTS:

- 100 g noodle soba.
- 100 g curly shredded broccoli.
- Sesame Oil 2 tsp.
- Two lean breasts of meat, skin off, cut into thin pieces.
- 25 g fresh ginger portion, peeled and cut into matching rods.
- One hot, required, thin-sliced pepper
- Handful sprouting of Brussels, sliced into pieces.
- One tbsp of soy sauce low sodium
- 2 tbsp rice wine or vinegar with white wine
- One lime juice and zest.

INSTRUCTIONS:

1. Cook the noodles according to the directions for packaging, then drain and set aside. In the meantime, heat a large wok or frying pan and add the kale with a good splash of water and cook for 1-2 minutes until wild, with the remaining snap, then cool under running water to keep the color.
2. Add half the oil and cook the chicken strips until browned, then cut and put differently. Heat the remaining oil until it is a little softened, cook the ginger, pepper and sprout. Remove the poultry and kale and add the noodles.
3. Tip on the soy, rice wine, lime zest and juice along with enough water to make a sauce that adheres to ingredients, serve straight away.

21. CHICKEN, BROCCOLI AND BEETROOT SALAD WITH AVOCADO PESTO

This superfood supper is filled with ingredients to strengthen the body, including red onion, rapeseed oil, nigella seeds, walnuts, and lemon

INGREDIENTS:

- Thin-strained broccoli 250gm.
- Rapeseed oil 2 tsp.
- Three skinless breasts of chicken.
- One red thinly sliced onion.
- Watercress 100g bag.
- Two raw beetroots (about 175 g), peeled
- Seeds of nigella 1 tsp.
- For pesto avocado.
- Small basil bag.
- One Avocado.
- Smashed 1/2 garlic cloves
- Crumbled 25 g walnut pieces
- Rapeseed oil 1 tbsp.
- One lemon juice and zest.

INSTRUCTIONS:

1. Bring to a boil a wide pan of water, add the broccoli and cook for 2 minutes. Drain, then under cool water to clean. Heat a griddle plate, toss the broccoli for 2-3 mins in 1/2 tsp of the rapeseed oil and griddle, rotating, until a little charred. Put aside to freshen up. Brush the remaining oil and season into the bird. Griddle on either side for 3-4 minutes or until it is cooked clean. Leave to cool, then break into chunky bits or shred them.

2. Insert the pesto next. Choose the basil leaves, then set aside a few of them to cover the salad. Place the remainder inside a food processor's little pot. Scoop the avocado flesh and add the garlic, walnuts, sugar, 1 tbsp lemon juice, 2-3 tbsp of cold water and some seasoning to the food processor. Blitz until flat, then move to a small serving platter. Pour the remainder of the lemon juice

over the sliced onions, and leave for a few minutes.

3. Put the watercress onto a broad bowl. Toss the broccoli and onion, along with the lemon juice in which they were soaked. Top up the beetroot, but don't combine it with the chicken. Disperse the reserved basil leaves, lemon zest and nigella seeds and serve with pesto avocado.

22. KALE WITH LEMON TAHINI DRESSING

A simple and easy side dish stir-fried on the kale. Drizzle over a glug of the lemon tahini dressing to make your greens flavorful and new

INGREDIENTS:

- One lemon juice (about 3 tbsp)
- Smashed One garlic clove.
- Tahini 50 g.
- One cup of olive oil.
- Kale 200 g.

INSTRUCTIONS:

1. Next, button it up. In a tiny cup, apply the lemon juice, garlic, tahini and 50ml of cool water. Mix well to shape a loose dressing and to taste the season. (Don't panic if it gets divided at first – it should fall back when you mix it).
2. Heat the oil in a big pot and stir-fry the kale for 3 minutes. Attach half the dressing to the saucepan and cook for 30 secs. Move the remaining dressing to a serving bowl and drizzle over.

23. THE SIRTFOOD DIET'S CORONATION CHICKEN SALAD

INGREDIENTS:

- 75 g Yogurt Regular
- 1/4th lemon water
- One tablespoon, chopped, coriander
- One tablespoon. Turmeric field
- 1/2 tablespoon of mild curry powder
- 100 g Cooked breast chicken, sliced into bite-size
- 6 Half walnut, finely minced
- 1 Date of Medjool, thinly cut
- 20 g Dice of red onion
- 1 Chili bird's eye
- Rocket 40 grams, for eating

INSTRUCTIONS:

1. In a mug, mix the yogurt, lemon juice, coriander and spices. Attach the remainder of the ingredients and put on a rocket pad.

24. THE SIRTFOOD DIET'S BUNLESS BEEF BURGERS WITH ALL THE TRIMMINGS

INGREDIENTS:

- 125 g of lean minced beef (5% fat)
- 15 g of red, finely diced onion.
- One tablespoon of Parsley, diced thinly
- One tablespoon of Extra virgin Olive oil
- Sweet potatoes 150 g
- One tablespoon of Olive oil super-pure
- One tablespoon of clean rosemary
- 1 Clove of garlic, unpeeled
- 10 gm Cheese cheddar, cut or grated
- 150 g red, ring-sliced onion
- 30 gm Sliced tomato
- Missile weighing 10 gm
- One (optional) Gherkin

INSTRUCTIONS:

1. Heat the oven up to 220oC / gas 7
2. Start by making some fries. Peel and shape into 1 cm thick chips the sweet potato. Attach the olive oil, rosemary and garlic clove to them. Place on a baking sheet and fry for 30 minutes, until smooth and crisp.
3. For the steak, combine the ground beef with the onion and the parsley. Unless you have pastry cutters, you may be able to shape your burger with the biggest pastry cutter in the package, otherwise, use your hands to create only a decent patty.
4. Heat the frying pan over medium heat, add the oil, put the burger on one side of the pan and rings the onion on the other side. Cook the burger on each side for 6 minutes, to ensure it is cooked through. When fried to your taste, fry the onion rings.
5. Top with the cheese and red onion when the burger is cooked and place it in a hot oven for a minute to melt. Remove the tomato, rocket and gherkin and top it with. Serve with some fries.

25. THE SIRTFOOD DIET'S CHICKEN SKEWERS WITH SATAY SAUCE

INGREDIENTS:

- 150 g of chicken breast, cut into pieces.
- One tablespoon terrestrial turmeric.
- 1/2 tablespoon live oil is particularly virgin.
- Buckwheat: 50 g.
- Kale 30 g, stalks removed and trimmed.
- 30 gm Sliced celery.
- Four half walnut, sliced, to garnish.
- 20 g diced red onion
- One Clove of garlic, minced
- One tablespoon olive oil is particularly virgin
- One tablespoon curried milk
- One tablespoon terrestrial turmeric
- Chicken stock: 50 ml
- Coconut milk: 150 ml
- 1tablespoon butter with walnut or peanut butter
- One tablespoon chopped Coriander

INSTRUCTIONS:

1. Mix the chicken with olive oil and turmeric and reserve to marinate-30 minutes to 1 hour is best, but just leave it as long as you can if you are short in time.
2. Cook the buckwheat and add the kale and celery to the last 5–7 minutes of the cooking time according to the package instructions. Hey, drain.
3. Heat the barbecue in a high setting.
4. Gently fry the red onion and garlic in the olive oil for 2-3 minutes until soft. Add the spices and cook for another minute. Add the stock and the coconut milk and bring to a boil, then add the walnut butter and stir. Reduce heat and simmer the sauce for 8-10 minutes or until creamy and rich.
5. As the sauce simmers, add the chicken to the skewers and place it under the hot grill for 10 minutes, turning it after 5 minutes.

6. To serve, stir the coriander in the sauce and pour over the
   skewers, then spread over the chopped walnuts.

26. THE SIRTFOOD DIET'S SMOKED SALMON OMELET

INGREDIENTS:

- Two eggs small
- 100 g Smoked, cut salmon
- 1/2 dc. Capers.-Capers
- 10 g of a rocket, cut
- One tablespoon chopped Parsley
- One tablespoon olive oil extra virgin

INSTRUCTIONS:

1. Smash the eggs and whisk them into a tub. Stir in the salmon, capers, rockets, and Persil.
2. In a non-stick oven, heat the olive oil till it is dry, but not smoking. Attach the egg blend and push the blend around the pan using a spatula or fish slice until even. Reduce the heat and cook the omelet. Slide around the edges of the spatula and roll the omelet or fold it in half to serve.

27. THE SIRTFOOD DIET'S SHAKSHUKA

INGREDIENTS:

- One tablespoon of olive Oil Extra Virgin
- 40 gm of fine cut red onion
- One Garlic clove, thinly sliced
- Thirty grams of celery, chopped
- Chili 1 bird's eye, good cut
- One tablespoon cumin Groud
- One tablespoon turmeric – Field turmeric.
- One tablespoon paprika.
- 400 g Chopped tinned tomatoes
- 30 g Kale, trimmed stalks and cut roughly.
- One tablespoon Parsley captured.
- Two small eggs.

INSTRUCTIONS:

1. Heat over medium to low heat a small, deep-seated frying pan. Add the oil and fry for 1–2 minutes onion, garlic, celery, chili, and spices.
2. Add the tomatoes, then leave the sauce for 20 minutes to heat slowly, stirring periodically.

28. THE SIRTFOOD DIET'S DATE AND WALNUT PORRIDGE

INGREDIENTS:

- 50 g Strawberries, hulled
- 200 ml Milk or dairy-free alternative
- 35 g Buckwheat flakes
- One Medjool date, chopped
- One tsp. Walnut butter or four chopped walnut halves

INSTRUCTIONS:

1. Put the milk and the date in a saucepan, heat gently, then add the buckwheat flakes and cook until the porridge is the consistency you like.
2. Add the walnut butter or walnuts, stir in the strawberries and serve.
3. Mix in the kale and roast for another 5 minutes. When you thought the sauce is too deep, just apply a bit of water. Stir in the parsley, if your sauce has a good rich flavor.
4. Make two small sauce wells and spit each egg into them. Reduce heat to its lowest setting and use a lid or foil to cover the pan. Leave the eggs for 10–12 minutes to cook, where the whites should be firm while the yolks are still runny. Cook for an extra 3–4 minutes, if you like strong yolks. Serve right away- preferably straight from the jar.

29. THE SIRTFOOD DIET'S BRAISED PUY LENTILS

INGREDIENTS:

- 8 Cherry tomatoes halved
- 40 g Red onion, thinly sliced
- 2 tsp. Extra virgin olive oil
- 40 g Celery, thinly sliced
- 1 Garlic clove, finely chopped
- 1 tsp. Paprika
- 40 g Carrots, peeled and thinly sliced
- 1 tsp. Thyme (dry or fresh)
- 220 ml Vegetable stock
- 75 g Puy lentils
- 20 g Rocket
- 1 tbsp. Parsley, chopped
- 50 g Kale, roughly chopped

INSTRUCTIONS:

1. Heat up 120 ° C / gas 1/2. Heat your oven.
2. In a small roasting tin, place the tomatoes and roast in the oven for 35-45 minutes.
3. Heat the bowl over a medium-low flame. Stir the red Onion, garlic, celery and carotene in 1 teaspoon of olive oil, fry it for 1–2 minutes, until softened. Attach the paprika and thyme and cook for a minute.
4. Rinse the lenses and add them to the pot along with the stock in a finely mixed pan. Bring to boil, then raising heat and cook with a cloth on the saucepan for 20 minutes. Add a little water if the level drops too much and add a stir every 7 minutes.
5. Cook for another 10 minutes, add the kale. Stir in the pettles and roasted tomatoes when the lentils are cooked. Serve the remaining tablespoon with the olive oil with the racket. Serve.

30. THE SIRTFOOD DIET'S PRAWN ARRABBIATA

INGREDIENTS:

- 65 g Buckwheat pasta
- Raw or cooked prawns (Ideally king prawns)
- One tbsp of Extra virgin olive oil
- One Garlic clove, finely chopped
- 40 g Red onion, finely chopped
- 1 Bird's eye chili, finely chopped
- 30 g Celery, finely chopped
- 1 tsp. Dried mixed herbs
- 1 tsp. Extra virgin olive oil
- 400 g Tinned chopped tomatoes
- 2 tbsp. White wine (optional)
- 1 tbsp. Chopped parsley

INSTRUCTIONS:

1. Fry in oil for a half-low heat and for 1-2 minutes the onion, garlic, celery and chili and herbs. Turn the heat to moderate, add the wine for 1 minute and cook. Attach tomatoes and keep the sauce cooled for 20-30 minutes over medium-low heat until the sauce is nice and creamy. Just add a little water if you feel the sauce becomes too thick.
2. Carry a bowl of water to boil during cooking and cook the pasta as instructed by the packet. Drain the olive oil and hold in the pan until required when cooked to your taste.
3. Add raw creams to the sauce, cook for 3 to 4 minutes and then add the parsley until they have become rose and opaque, and serve. Bring the sauce to the boil and serve if you use cooked creams with parsley.
4. Add to the sauce cooked pasta, carefully yet gently mix and serve.

31. THE SIRTFOOD DIET'S TURMERIC BAKED SALMON

INGREDIENTS:

- One tsp. Ground turmeric
- One tsp. Extra virgin olive oil
- One tsp. Extra virgin olive oil
- 1/4 Juice of a lemon
- 60 g Tinned green lentils
- 40 g Red onion, finely chopped
- One Bird's eye chili, finely chopped
- One Garlic clove, finely chopped
- One tsp. Mild curry powder
- 150 gm Celery, cut into 2cm lengths
- 100 ml Chicken or vegetable stock
- 130 gm Tomato, cut into eight wedges
- Skinned Salmon
- One tbsp. Chopped parsley

INSTRUCTIONS:

1. Heat the oven to level 6 with gas / 200C.
2. Start with the celery spicy. Heat a pot over moderate to low heat, add the onion, garlic, ginger, chili, and celery to the olive oil.
3. Cook gently until soft and uncolored for about two to three minutes, then add the curry powder and start cooking for another minute.
4. Add the tomatoes and the lenses and gently cook for about 10 minutes. You may want to increase or reduce the cooking time according to how crunchy the celery is.
5. Mix turmeric, olive oil and lemon juice in the meantime. Cook for 8-10 minutes, place on a baking tray.
6. Finish by mixing the celery with the silk and serving with the salmon.

32. EASY PEASY CHICKEN CURRY

INGREDIENTS

- Three garlic cloves roughly chopped
- One red onion roughly chopped
- Two teaspoons garam masala
- 2 cm fresh ginger peeled and roughly chopped
- Two teaspoons ground turmeric
- Two teaspoons ground cumin
- One cinnamon stick optional
- One tbsp of olive oil
- Six cardamom pods optional
- One x 400ml tin coconut milk
- Eight boneless of chicken thighs, cut into bitesize chunks, or four chicken breasts.
- 200 gm of brown or basmati rice buckwheat to dish.
- Two tablespoons fresh coriander chopped (plus extra for garnish)

INSTRUCTIONS:

1. In the food processor, put the onion, garlic and ginger and lightning until the paste. Alternatively, chop these three ingredients thoroughly and continue as below, if you don't have one.
2. Stir in the paste with the garam massale, cumin and turmeric. Place aside. Set aside.
3. Placed in a big depth (ideally non-stick) 1 tablespoon of olive oil. For a minute, heat up the bowl, then add the chopped chicken thighs. Pour the chicken over high heat, and add to the curry paste. Turn it down for 2 minutes.
4. Let the chicken cook for 3 minutes in the paste and then add half the milk (200ml) and the cinnamon (if using) cardamom. Turn down and cook until the curried sauce is thick and delicious, and then let it simmer for 30 minutes.
5. Apply more coconut milk as the curry starts to heat, maybe you don't need anything, but if you want a much more clever curry, add the lot!

6. Make your accompaniment (snack/rice) and any side dishes during the cooking process.
7. When the curry is finished, add the sliced coriander and serve with sweet or rice and a good glass of chilled white wine, medium water immediately!

33. KING PRAWN STIR FRY WITH BUCKWHEAT NOODLES

INGREDIENTS:

- Two tablespoons extra virgin olive oil
- 300 g buckwheat/soba noodles try to get 100% buckwheat if you can
- Two sticks of celery sliced
- One red onion sliced thinly
- 100 g green beans chopped
- 100 g kale roughly chopped
- Three garlic cloves grated or finely chopped
- 3 cm ginger grated
- 600 g king prawns
- One bird's eye chili seeds/membranes removed and chopped finely (or more to taste)
- Two tablespoons tamari/soy sauce plus extra for serving
- Two tablespoons parsley chopped (or lovage if you can get it!)

INSTRUCTIONS:

1. Cook noodles for 3-5 minutes or until you like them. Rinse in cold water, wash. Drizzle over a little olive oil, mix together and hold.
2. Prepare remaining ingredients while the noodles are cooking.
3. Fry the red onion and celery in a broad wok or saucepan for 3 minutes in moderate heat in a mild olive oil and add the kale and green boobs and cook for three minutes in medium-high heat.
4. Remove heat and add ginger, garlic, chili and butter. Crumble for 2-3 minutes until crevasses are dry.
5. Add noodles, tamari/soy sauce, and cook 1-minute longer until the noodles are again dry. Strain and serve with parsley.

34. BAKED POTATOES WITH SPICY CHICKPEA STEW (VEGAN)

Spicy Chickpea Curry baked potatoes. Mexican mole kind meets North African tagine. It is amazingly amazing, makes a perfect top for baked pulp, as well as vegetarian, vegan, gluten-free and milk free. And the chocolate is there.

INGREDIENTS:

- Two tablespoons olive oil
- 4-6 baking potatoes pricked all over
- Four cloves garlic grated or crushed
- Two red onions finely chopped
- 2 cm ginger grated
- Two tablespoons cumin seeds
- ½ -two tsp of chili flakes depending on how hot you like things
- Splash of water
- Two tablespoons turmeric
- Two tsp unsweetened cocoa powder or cacao
- 2 x 400g tins chickpeas or kidney beans if you prefer, including the chickpea water, don't drain!
- Two yellow peppers or whatever color you prefer! chopped into bitesize pieces
- 2 x 400g tins chopped tomatoes
- Salt and pepper to taste optional
- Two tablespoons parsley plus extra for garnish
- Side salad optional

INSTRUCTIONS:

1. Preheat the oven to 200C, while all the ingredients can be prepared.
2. Put the baking potatoes in the oven when the oven is hot enough, and cook 1 hour or until they're finished as you want them. (If it's different from mine, feel free to use your usual baked potato method!)
3. Put olive oil and chopped red onion in an oven in a big broad

casserole once in the oven and gradually cook with the lid until the onion is tender, but not brown for 5 minutes.

4. Remove the lid and add the cumin, chili and garlic. Add the curds and a very small splash of water for another minute and cook for a minute, taking care not to let the pan dry enough and cook for a minute.

5. Add the tomatoes and cacao powder, chickpeas and yellow pepper, as well as chickpea juice. Bring to a boil, then cook 45 minutes on low heat until the sauce is thick and unctuous (but do not allow it to burn!). The stew will take place roughly with the potatoes.

6. Serve a skewer with a simple side salad on the baked Pommes of terracotta, and add 2 table cubs of parsley, salt and pepper if necessary.

35. KALE AND RED ONION DHAL WITH BUCKWHEAT (VEGAN)

Kale and Buckwheat Red Onion Dhal. This Kale and Red Onion Dhal are delicious and very nutritious with buckwheat that can be conveniently and quickly processed without gluten OR milk. Suitable for vegetarians or vegan.

INGREDIENTS:

- One small red onion sliced
- One tablespoon olive oil
- 2 cm ginger grated
- Three garlic cloves grated or crushed
- Two teaspoons turmeric
- One bird's eye chili deseeded and finely chopped (more if you like things hot!)
- 160 g red lentils
- Two teaspoons garam masala
- 200 ml of water
- 400 ml of coconut milk
- 160 g buckwheat or brown rice
- 100 g kale or spinach would be a great alternative

INSTRUCTIONS:

1. In a deep, broad casserole, put the olive oil and add onion sliced. Cook in low heat and the lid will be softened for 5 minutes.
2. Add garlic, chili-ginger and cook for another 1 minute.
3. Attach the turmeric and a sprinkling of water to the garam masala, and cook for another 1 minute.
4. Apply the red lens, chocolate milk and 200 ml water (just half of the cocoa milk can be filled with water and tipped into the cup).
5. Mix everything carefully and cook over low heat with the lid for 20 minutes. Extract from time to time, add some more water if the dhal sticks.
6. Stir and remove your cap, add kale after 20 minutes (1-2 minutes if you're wearing spinach instead!); cook for another 5 minutes.
7. Put buckwheat in a medium pot and add plenty of boiling water

about 15 minutes before the curry is ready. Return the water to the boil again and cook 10 minutes (or a little longer if it is softer. Drain the buckwheat into a sieve and use the dhal.

36. THE SIRTFOOD DIET GREEN JUICE SALAD

This salad includes two more Sirt, walnuts and olive oil with the same ingredients as the green drink, as well as the orange Sirt. Superb and simple to construct.

INGREDIENTS:

- 1 cm of ginger grated
- Juice of ½ lemon
- One tablespoon olive oil
- Salt and pepper to taste
- One handful rocket
- Two handfuls kale sliced
- Two celery sticks sliced
- One tablespoon parsley
- Six walnut halves
- ½ green apple sliced

INSTRUCTIONS:

1. In a jam container, add the lemon juice, ginger, salt, pumice and olive oil.
2. In a large cup, place the kale and pour over the dressing. Wear the dressing for 1 minute to rub into the kale.
3. Add the other ingredients and thoroughly blend together.

37. THE SIRTFOOD DIET GREEN JUICE

The green juice is full of nutrient rich Sirt foods, which are taken from the recipes in the Sirtfood Diet. This is ideal for those who want to get healthy, important to the Sirtfood Diet.

INGREDIENTS:

- 30 g rocket
- 75 g kale
- 5 g parsley
- ½ green apple
- Two celery sticks
- Juice of ½ lemon
- 1 cm ginger
- ½ teaspoon matcha green tea

INSTRUCTIONS:

1. Juice all the ingredients except the citrus and green tea matcha.
2. Hand in the green juice squeeze the lemon juice
3. Mix in a glass a tiny amount and add a little green juice. Through the bottle and add with the rest of the green juice.
4. Save or drink immediately.

38. TURMERIC CHICKEN & KALE SALAD
WITH HONEY LIME DRESSING

Notes: *Dress the salad ten minutes before serving if prepared in advance. Beef small, chopped creeping prawns and fish can replace chicken. Vegetarians may use mushrooms or quinoa cooked.*

INGREDIENTS:

For the chicken

- ½ medium brown onion, diced
- One tsp ghee or 1 tbsp of coconut oil
- One large garlic clove should be finely diced
- 250-300 g / 9 oz. chicken mince or diced up chicken thighs
- One teaspoon lime zest
- One teaspoon turmeric powder
- ½ teaspoon salt + pepper
- juice of ½ lime

For the salad

- Two tablespoons pumpkin seeds (pepitas)
- Six broccolini stalks or 2 cups of broccoli florets
- ½ avocado, sliced
- Three large kale leaves stem removed and chopped
- A handful of fresh parsley leaves, chopped
- A handful of fresh coriander leaves, chopped

For the dressing

- One small garlic clove, finely diced or grated
- Three tablespoons lime juice
- Three tablespoons extra-virgin olive oil (I used one tablespoon avocado oil and * 2 tablespoons EVO)
- One teaspoon raw honey
- Three tablespoons extra-virgin olive oil (I used one tablespoon avocado oil and * 2 tablespoons EVO)

- ½ teaspoon sea salt and pepper
- ½ teaspoon wholegrain or Dijon mustard

INSTRUCTIONS:

1. In a small frying pan over medium to high flame, flame ghee or coconut oil. Add onion and sauté 4-5 minutes, until golden, at medium heat. Remove the chicken thin and garlic and brush over medium-high heat for 2-3 minutes and then separate.
2. Mix and cook turmeric, lime zest, lime juice, salt and pepper for a further 3-4 minutes. Stir regularly. Put aside the cooked thin.
3. Put a small pot of water to boil while the chicken is cooking. Stir and cook the broccolini for 2 minutes. Rince and cut into 3-4 pieces, each under cold water.
4. Stirring regularly to avoid burning, add pumpkin seeds into the frypan from the chicken and toast over medium heat for 2 minutes. A little salt season. Season. Place aside. Set aside. Pure seeds from pumpkin are also appropriate for use.
5. Place the sliced kale in a salad bowl and pipe over the sandwich. Place your hands on the dressing and rub the egg. The sluts are smooth – they are partially "fried" – like citrus juice to fish or beef carpaccio. Bring in finally the fried rice, broccolini, new herbs, seeds of pumpkin and avocado.

39. BUCKWHEAT NOODLES WITH CHICKEN KALE & MISO DRESSING

INGREDIENTS:

For the noodles

- 2-3 pound of kale leaves (roughly cut out of the stem)
- Buckwheat noodles 150 g/5 oz (100% buckwheat, no wheat)
- 3-4 shiitake champagne, cut. Cut.
- One tablespoon of ghee or coconut oil
- One brown, fine-diced onion
- Chicken, sliced or diced one free-range media breast.
- One long, thinly sliced red chill (seeds inside or out, according to how hot you like)
- Two common, finely diced garlic cloves
- Tamari sauce with 2-3 teaspoons (gluten-free)
- For the miso dressing
- One tablespoon Tamari sauce
- 1½ tablespoon fresh organic miso
- One tablespoon lemon or lime juice
- One tablespoon extra-virgin olive oil
- One teaspoon sesame oil (optional)

INSTRUCTIONS:

1. Put to boil a medium water cup. Attach the kale and cook until slightly diluted, for 1 minute. Remove, save the water and bring it to the boil again. Drain it. Fill the soba noodles and cook (usually approximately 5 minutes) according to package directions. Rinse and set aside under cold water.
2. Meanwhile, fry the shiitake champignon for 2-3 minutes with a little ghee or coconut oil (around a teaspoon), until nicely browned on either side. Pour in salt and set aside. Sprinkle.
3. Heat coconut oil or ghee over medium-high heat in the same frying saucepan
4. Pour into onion or chili and add chicken parts for 2-3 minutes. Cook over medium heat five minutes, stirring a few times, then

add a small amount of garlic, tamari sauce, and tea. Cook for another 2-3 minutes, frequently mix until chicken is finished.

5. Add the chicken noodle and soba, and cook up through the food.
6. At the very end of cooking, blend the miso dressing and twinkling over the noodles to keep all of these beneficial probiotics alive.

40. CHOC CHIP GRANOLA-SIRTFOOD RECIPES

Breakfast cake! Make sure to serve you plenty of SIRTs with a cup of green tea. If you want, you can substitute the rice malt syrup with maple syrup.

INGREDIENTS:

- 50g pecans, chopped roughly
- 200g jumbo oats
- 20g butter
- 3 tbsp light olive oil
- 2 tbsp rice malt syrup
- 1 tbsp dark brown sugar
- dark chocolate chips
- 60g good-quality (70%)

INSTRUCTIONS

1. Preheat oven to 140 ° C (gas 3). Preheat oven to 160 ° C. Line a major bakery with a sheet of silicone or pastry.
2. In a large tub, mix oats and pecans. Heat olive oil, butter, brown sugar and rice malt syrup gently in a small, non-stick pot until butter melts and the sugar and syrup are dissolved. Don't authorize boiling. Pour the syrup over the oats and mix until full coverage of the oats is complete.
3. Spread the granola over the bakery and spread into the corners.
4. Having mixture clumps with distance instead of spreading. Twenty minutes in the oven until the edges are light brown. Take out of the oven and allow the tray to refresh completely.
5. Separate with your fingertips and then blend the chocolate with any large bumps in a tray when it's cold. Grab or pour the granola into a bowl or container airtight. At least two weeks the granola will stay.

41. BAKED SALMON SALAD WITH CREAMY MINT DRESSING-SIRTFOOD RECIPES

It is easy to roast the salmon in the oven.

INGREDIENTS:

- 40g mixed salad leaves
- One salmon fillet (130g)
- Two radishes, trimmed and thinly sliced
- 40g young spinach leaves
- Two spring onions, trimmed and sliced
- 5cm piece (50g) cucumber, cut into chunks
- One small handful (10g) parsley, roughly chopped

For the dressing:

- One tablespoon natural yogurt
- One tablespoon low-fat mayonnaise
- Two leaves mint, finely chopped
- One tablespoon rice vinegar
- Salt and freshly ground black pepper

INSTRUCTIONS:

1. Preheat the oven to 200oC (fan/gas six at a temperature of 180oC).
2. Through the salmon fillet on a baker and bake until cooked for 16-18 minutes. Remove and set aside from the oven. The salmon in the salad is just as nice warm or cold. If your salmon has meat, just cook the skin down and separate it from the skin with a fish slice. When fried, it will slide quickly.
3. Mix the mayonnaise, yogurt and rice vinegar together in a small bowl and add the leaves and salt and pepper with the mixture to allow the aromas to develop for at least 5 minutes.
4. Settle the salad leaves and spinach with radishes, cucumber, ointments of the spring and pets on the serving plate and top. Place the cooked salmon on the salad and dress up.

42. FRAGRANT ASIAN HOTPOT-SIRTFOOD RECIPES

INGREDIENTS:

- One star anise, crushed (or 1/4 tsp ground anise)
- 1 tsp tomato purée
- Small handful (1Og) coriander, stalks finely chopped
- Small handful (10g) parsley, stalks finely chopped
- 1/2 carrot, peeled and cut into matchsticks
- 50gm beansprouts
- 50gm broccoli, cut into small florets
- 100gm firm tofu, chopped
- 100gm raw tiger prawns
- 50g rice noodles, cooked according to packet
- 20g sushi ginger, chopped
- 50g cooked water chestnuts, drained
- 1 tbsp good-quality miso paste

INSTRUCTIONS:

1. Put in a bread pan and simmer for 10 minutes, the stirring tomato, star anise, petty stalks, coriander stalks and lime juice.
2. Add carrot, broccoli, creeping pies, tofu, chestnuts and water noodles and gently cook until creeping is finished. Stir the sushi ginger and miso paste from the heat. Stir.
3. Serve with pins and coriander leaves.

43. LAMB, BUTTERNUT SQUASH AND DATE TAGINE

Unbelievable dry Moroccan spices make this balanced day ideal for icy fall and winter days. For an extra health kick, serve with buckwheat!

INGREDIENTS:

- One red onion, sliced
- Two tablespoons olive oil
- Three garlic cloves, grated or crushed
- 2cm ginger, grated
- Two teaspoons cumin seeds
- One teaspoon chili flakes (or to taste)
- Two teaspoons ground turmeric
- One cinnamon stick
- ½ teaspoon salt
- 800g lamb neck fillet, cut into 2cm chunks
- 500g butternut squash, chopped into 1cm cubes
- 400g tin chopped tomatoes, plus half a can of water
- Two tablespoons fresh coriander (plus extra for garnish)
- 400g tin chickpeas, drained
- Buckwheat, couscous, flatbreads or rice to serve

INSTRUCTIONS:

1. Preheat to 140C for your oven
2. Drizzle in a large ovenproof casserole or cast casserole dish around two cubic cubes of olive oil. Slice onion and heat until the onions are smooth but not browned, with a cover on for about 5 minutes.
3. Ginger, chili, cumin, cinnamon, and turmeric are added to the grilled garlic. Cover well and cook with the lid for another 1 minute. If it gets too dry, add a sprinkle of water.
4. Add next chunks of lamb. Add the butter, minced dates and tomato and a further half a can of water (100-200mL) to cover the meat in the onions and Spices. Mix well.
5. Bring the tagine to a simmer, then place on the cover and place 1 hour and 15 minutes in your pre-heated oven.

6. Add chopped butternut squash and drained chickpeas thirty minutes prior to the end of the cooking period. Put the cover on and back in the oven for the remaining 30 minutes of the preparation, bringing it together.
7. Turn off the oven and mix with chopped coriander when tagine is finished. Serve with couscous, basmati or buckwheat.

Notes: If you don't own an ovenproof casserole or iron cast casserole dish, just bake the tagine in an ordinary bowl until it's in the oven and transfer it to an ordinary saucer before putting the tagine in the oven. Add an additional five minutes to cook to give more room to heat in the saucepan.

44. PRAWN ARRABBIATA-SIRTFOOD RECIPES

INGREDIENTS:

- 65 g of sweetheart pasta.
- 125-150 g Raw or cooked crevices (ideally king crevices)
- For sauce arrabbiata.
- Extra virgin olive oil 1 tbsp extra.
- One clove of garlic, finely cut.
- 40 g of finely sliced red onion.
- 1 Chili eye bird, smoothly chopped.
- Thirty g celery, thinly sliced.
- 1 tsp Olive Oil Extra Virgin.
- 1 tsp Mixed herbs dried.
- 400 g Tinned tomatoes sliced.
- 2 tbsp of white (optional) wine.
- 1 tbsp Chopped parsley

INSTRUCTIONS:

- Fry in oil for a half-low heat and for 1-2 minutes the onion, garlic, celery and chili and herbs. Switch the heat to mild, add the wine for 1 minute and cook. Add tomatoes and keep the sauce cooled for 20-30 minutes over medium-low heat until the sauce is good and thick. Just add a little water if you feel the sauce becomes too thick.
- Bring a bowl of water to boil during cooking and cook the pasta as directed by the packet. Drain the olive oil and keep in the pan until necessary when cooked to your liking.
- Add raw creams to the sauce, cook for 3 to 4 minutes and then add the parsley until they have become rose and opaque, and serve. Carry the sauce to the boil and drink whether you use boiled creams with parsley.
- Add to the sauce cooked pasta, carefully but gently mix and serve.

45. TURMERIC BAKED SALMON-SIRTFOOD RECIPES

INGREDIENTS:

- 1 tsp Olive oil extra virgin.
- Skinned salmon between 125-150 g.
- 1/4 Lemon Juice.
- 1 tsp of turmeric grain.
- 1 tsp Olive oil extra virgin.
- For the celery spicy.
- Around 60 g Green lentils.
- Around 40 g of red, finely chopped onion.
- 1 cm of fresh, finely chopped ginger.
- 1 Clove of garlic, finely minced.
- Cut into 2 cm lengths about 150 g Celery.
- 1 Chili of the bird's eye, finely chopped.130 g Tomato, cut into eight wedges
- 1 tsp Mild curry powder
- 1 tbsp Chopped parsley
- 100 ml Chicken or vegetable stock

INSTRUCTIONS:

1. Heat the furnace to mark 200C / gas 6.
2. The hot celery ends. Cover the pot with olive oil, then add onion, garlic, ginger, chili and celery over low-medium flame. Fritter gently for 2 to 3 minutes and then apply the curry powder and cook for another minute, until softer but not marked.
3. Then add the tomatoes and the lenses and gently cook for 10 minutes. You might want to raise or lower the cooking time according to how crunchy the celery is.
4. Mix the turmeric, butter and lemon juice in the meantime, then roll the salmon over it.
5. Cook 8-10 minutes, then placed on the baking tray.
6. Stir in celery and serve with the salmon in order to finish.

46. CORONATION CHICKEN SALAD

INGREDIENTS:

- Juice of 1/4 of a lemon
- 75 g Natural yogurt
- One tablespoon ground turmeric
- One tablespoon Coriander, chopped
- 100 g Cooked chicken breast, cut into bite-sized pieces
- 1/2 tsp Mild curry powder
- 1 Medjool date, finely chopped
- 6 Walnut halves, finely chopped
- 1 Bird's eye chili
- 20 g Red onion, diced
- 40 g Rocket, to serve

INSTRUCTION:

1. In a cup mix the milk, the orange water, coriander and the spices
2. Serve on a rocket bed, adding all remaining ingredients.

47. BAKED POTATOES WITH SPICY CHICKPEA STEW-SIRTFOOD RECIPES

Sort of Mexican Mole, this Hot STEW TREE is amazingly wonderful and offers an outstanding top topping with baked potatoes plus vegetarian, organic and gluten-free, milk-free. And chocolate is in it.

INGREDIENTS:

- Two tablespoons olive oil
- 4-6 baking potatoes, pricked all over
- Four cloves garlic, grated or crushed
- Two red onions, finely chopped
- ½ -2 teaspoons chili flakes (depending on how hot you like things)
- 2cm ginger, grated
- Two tbsp of turmeric
- Two tbsp of cumin seeds
- 2 x 400g tins chopped tomatoes
- Splash of water
- 2 x 400 g tins of chickpeas (or kidney beans if you prefer) also DON'T DRAIN chickpea water!!
- Two tablespoons unsweetened cocoa powder (or cacao)
- Two tablespoons parsley plus extra for garnish
- Salt and pepper to taste (optional)
- Two yellow peppers (or whatever color you prefer!), chopped into bitesize pieces
- Side salad (optional)

INSTRUCTIONS:

1. Preheat the oven to 200C, when all the supplies can be packed.
2. Place the baking potatoes in the oven when the oven is high enough, and cook 1 hour or until they're cooked as you want them.
3. Put olive oil and sliced red onion in an oven in a big broad casserole once in the oven and gradually cook with the cover until the onion is tender, but not brown for 5 minutes.
4. Remove the cover and apply the cumin, chili and garlic. Add the

curds and a very tiny splash of water for another minute and cook for a minute, take care not to make the pan hot sufficiently cook for a minute.

5. Introduce the tomatoes and cacao powder, chickpeas and yellow pepper, as well as chickpea juice. Bring to a boil, then cook 45 minutes on low heat until the sauce is thick and unctuous (but do not cause it to burn!). The stew will take place roughly with the potatoes.

6. Put a skewer on the baked potatoes, with a basic side salad, and then apply the two teaspoons of parsley and salt and pepper if you want.

48. GRAPE AND MELON JUICE-SIRTFOOD RECIPES

INGREDIENTS:

- 1/2 cucumber, peel if necessary, halving, scraping seeds and roughing.
- 30 g youthful spinach leaves, removed stalks.
- 100 g red grapes without seeds
- 100 g of melon, washed, wished and cut cantaloupe.

INSTRUCTION:

1. In a juicer or blender, mix together until smooth.

49. KALE AND RED ONION DHAL WITH BUCKWHEAT

This very Kale and Red Onion Dhal are delicious and very healthy with buckwheat, which can be processed easily and quickly without gluten, oil, vegetarian or vegan.

INGREDIENTS:

- One small red onion, sliced
- One tablespoon olive oil
- 2 cm ginger, grated
- Three garlic cloves, grated or crushed
- Two teaspoons turmeric
- One bird eye chili, deseeded and finely chopped (more if you like things hot!)
- 160g red lentils
- Two teaspoons garam masala
- 200ml water
- 400ml coconut milk
- 160g buckwheat (or brown rice)
- 100g kale (or spinach would be a great alternative)

INSTRUCTIONS:

1. In a broad, deep casserole, apply the olive oil and dice the onion. Cook in low temperatures with the lid softened for 5 minutes.
2. Add 1 minute of garlic, ginger and chili, and fry.
3. Apply turmeric, garam masala and water splash and cook 1 minute more.
4. Fill in red glasses, cocoon milk and 200ml of water by half the cocoon milk may be loaded with water and tipped into the bowl.
5. Thoroughly mix and cook over medium heat with the cover for 20 minutes. Remove from time to time; add a little more water when the dhal stays.
6. Attach the kale and whisk carefully.
7. Cook for another 5 minutes after 20 minutes (1-2 minutes if instead of using spinach!)
8. Put buckwheat in a medium pot and add plenty of boiling water

about 15 minutes before the curry is finished.
9. Take your buckwheat back to the boil and cook it for 10 minutes, or for a little bit longer if you like your softer buckwheat.

50. CHARGRILLED BEEF WITH A RED WINE JUS, ONION RINGS, GARLIC KALE AND HERB ROASTED POTATOES

INGREDIENTS:

- One tablespoon extra virgin olive oil
- 100g potatoes, peeled and cut into 2cm dice
- 50g red onion, sliced into rings
- 5g parsley, finely chopped
- One garlic clove, finely chopped
- 50g kale, sliced
- 40ml red wine
- 120–150g x 3.5cm-thick beef fillet steak or 2cm-thick sirloin steak
- 1 tsp tomato purée
- 150ml beef stock
- 1 tsp cornflour, dissolved in 1 tbsp water

INSTRUCTIONS:

1. Oven power to 220 ° C / gas 7.
2. Place the potatoes in a boiling pot and then drain for 4–5 minutes and put back to boil. In a roasting pan, apply one tablespoon of olive oil and roast 35-45 minutes in the hot oven. Placed the potatoes in order to ensure an even cooking per 10 minutes. Sprinkle the chopped Persil and mix well when cooked from the oven.
3. Fry onion for 5 to 7 minutes in one teaspoon of oil until soft and beautifully caramelized over medium heat. Keep dry.
4. Keeping it warm. Steam the kale and drain for about 2-3 minutes. Cook the goat softly, but not colored, in 1/2 teaspoon of oil for 1 minute. Attach the kale and brown before tender for another 1–2 minutes. Live wet. Remain dry.
5. Heat a high-heat oven-proof frying pan to smoke. Cook the meat in 1/2 teaspoon of oil and mix in the heated bowl over medium-high flame, if you prefer your beef. If you want to use the beef mild, stitch the meat and move the bowl to a 220oC / gas seven

furnace, such that the cooking may be done for the specified periods.

6. Take the meat out of the pot and put it aside. To collect any residue of meat, add wine to the hot pot. Bubble with a balanced taste to slash the wine by half.
7. Attach the pan to the stroked bowl, the tomato puree and the cornflour paste and thicken the sauce until you are of the perfect consistency. Eat the carrots, onions, onion rings and red sauce in the relaxed steak juice and eat.

51. KALE AND BLACKCURRANT SMOOTHIE

INGREDIENTS:

- One cup freshly made green tea
- 2 tsp honey
- One ripe banana
- Ten baby kale leaves stalk removed
- Six ice cubes
- 40 g blackcurrants, washed and stalks removed

INSTRUCTIONS:

1. Extract the honey until it is absorbed in the dry, green tea. Whisper in a mixer all ingredients into a fast processor. Serve right now.

52. BUCKWHEAT PASTA SALAD

INSTRUCTIONS:

- large handful of rocket
- 50g buckwheat pasta(cooked according to the packet instructions)Sirtfood recipes
- Eight cherry tomatoes halved
- A small handful of basil leaves
- Ten olives
- 1/2 avocado, diced
- 20g pine nuts
- 1 tbsp extra virgin olive oil

INSTRUCTIONS:

1. Mix all ingredients gently with the exception of the pine nut, and then arrange them on a plate or in a bowl.

53. GREEK SALAD SKEWERS

INGREDIENTS:

- Eight large black olives
- Two wooden skewers, soaked in water for 30 minutes before use
- One yellow pepper, cut into eight squares
- Eight cherry tomatoes
- 100g (about 10cm) cucumber, cut into four slices and halved
- ½ red onion, cut in half and separated into eight pieces
- 100g feta, cut into eight cubes

For the dressing:

- Juice of ½ lemon
- 1 tbsp extra virgin olive oil
- ½ clove garlic, peeled and crushed
- 1 tsp balsamic vinegar
- Few oregano seeds, thinly sliced.
-   Few basil leaves, thinly caught (or 1/2 tsp of drying, oregano and basil).
- Salt and black pepper seasoning.

INSTRUCTIONS:

1. Thread per skewer in order with the ingredients in the salad: olive, tomato, red onion, cucumber, cucumber, basil, garlic, red onion, pepper, feta. Thinning the skewer in the order with the salad ingredients
2. In a small pot, put all the dressing components and combine them thoroughly together. Verse the skewers around.

54. KALE, EDAMAME AND TOFU CURRY

INGREDIENTS:

- A big onion, cut.
- One tbsp of rapeseed oil
- A big, fresh, peeled and grated thumb (7 cm).
- Four garlic cloves, peeled and rubbing.
- Taste for 1/2 tsp of turmeric on the ground.
- A red chili that is wanted and slimly cut.1 tsp paprika
- 1/4 tsp cayenne pepper
- 1 tsp salt
- 1/2 tsp ground cumin
- One liter boiling water
- 250g dried red lentils
- 200g firm tofu, chopped into cubes
- 50g frozen soya edamame beans
- Juice of 1 lime
- Two tomatoes, roughly chopped
- 200g kale leaves stalk removed and torn

INSTRUCTIONS

1. Placed the oil in a heavy-bottom pan over the low-medium sun
2. Attach the onion and cook for 5 minutes before inserting the garlic, ginger and chili, and cook for another 2 minutes.
3. Remove the chili, cayenne, paprika, cumin and oil. Swirl once before inserting the red lentils and swirl again.
4. Pour in boiling water and simmer for 10 minutes, then rising the heat and cook for another 20-30 minutes before the curry has a deep 'porridge' consistency.
5. Add the rice, tofu and tomatoes and simmer for another 5 minutes. Add the lime juice and the kale leaves, then cook until the kale is soft.

55. CHOCOLATE CUPCAKES WITH MATCHA ICING

INGREDIENTS:

- 200 g of caster sugar.
- 150 g flour self-raising.
- Salt with 1/2 tsp.
- Cocoa 60 g.
- Dairy 120ml.
- Fine espresso coffee with 1/2 tsp, decaf if preferred
- 50ml vegetable oil
- ½ tsp vanilla extract
- 120ml boiling water
- One egg

For the icing:

- 50g icing sugar
- 50g butter, at room temperature
- ½ tsp vanilla bean paste
- 1 tbsp matcha green tea powder
- 50g soft cream cheese

INSTRUCTIONS:

1. Preheat the oven to a fan of 180C/160C, cover a cupcake tray with a paper or silicone cake shell.
2. Place the rice, sugar, chocolate, salt and espresso powder in a large bowl and blend thoroughly.
3. Apply the cream, vanilla extract, vegetable oil and egg to the dry ingredients and use an electric mixer until well mixed. Carefully dump gradually in the boiling water and pump at low speed before fully mixed.
4. Using high speed to beat for another minute and attach fuel to the pump. The dough is even more oily than the normal cake blend. Have faith; it's going to taste amazing!
5. Popular the batter equally between the cake cases. Each case of a cake will not be more than 3/4 whole. Bake in the oven for 15-18 minutes before the mixture has been tapped out. Remove from

the oven and allow it to cool completely before icing.
6. Mix the butter and icing sugar together until it is light and creamy. Add the matcha powder and vanilla, stir again. Attach the cream cheese and beat until smooth. Pipe or spray it over the cakes.

CONCLUSION

The Sirtfood Diet, created by nutritionists Aidan Goggins and Glen Matten, is the latest nutrition pattern to sweep the world, and the creators claim that it works to activate the "lean gene" of your body. The diet is a two-part approach and focuses on consuming foods rich in sirtuin, as well as calorie restriction.

Sirtuins are a group of seven proteins that protect our cells in the body from dying or being inflamed due to disease, explains nutritionist Michele, adding that research has also found that proteins can help regulate your metabolism, increase muscle and burn. Vet. polyphenols, Michele says, are micronutrients packed with antioxidants that have been found to improve digestion and neurodegenerative and cardiovascular diseases.

To begin dieting, participants should follow a two-week plan, which includes the reduction of calorie consumption and the consumption of "green sirt food" juices. "During the first week, you will limit [calorie] intake to 1,000 calories, which includes consuming three sirtfood-green juices and one meal rich in sirtfood per day," Michele shares. "The next week, she raises her intake to 1,500 calories a day and eats two food-rich meals and two green juices."

In the long run, no specific diet exists, but a high-nutritional diet plan is recommended, along with incorporating the green juices that are characteristic of the diet. The creators of the diet claim that the diet will lead to rapid weight loss while retaining muscle and mass and protecting you from chronic illnesses.

Do Not Go Yet; One Last Thing to Do

If you enjoyed this book or found it useful, I would be very grateful if you would post a short review on Amazon. Your support really does make a difference, and I read all the reviews personally so I can get your feedback and make this book even better.

Thanks again for your support!

9 798728 840145